MEDICAL/MORAL PROBLEMS

Medical/Moral Problems

Edited by
Robert Heyer

PAULIST PRESS
New York/Ramsey/Toronto

Art and Design: Gloria Ortíz

Library of Congress
Catalog Card Number: 77-83556

ISBN: 0-8091-2058-5

Published by Paulist Press
Editorial Office: 1865 Broadway, N.Y., N.Y. 10023
Business Office: 545 Island Rd., Ramsey, N.J. 07446

Printed and bound in the United States of America

CONTENTS

EUNICE KENNEDY SHRIVER

THE CHALLENGE OF THE

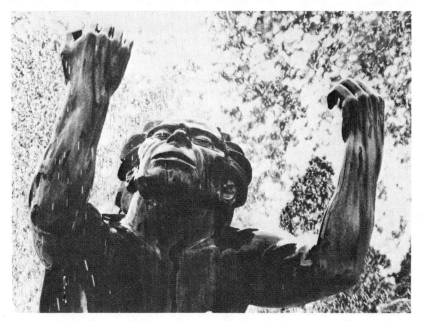

MENTALLY RETARDED

In the 1970's there are new and awesome challenges in the field of mental retardation.

The new challenges are: How can we make sure that the mentally retarded people in our midst can be guaranteed their human rights? How can we make sure that *their* right to life, liberty and the pursuit of happiness are protected? How can we make sure that they receive the education they deserve, the health treatment they deserve and the legal assistance they deserve?

These are the principal challenges of the future. To meet those challenges, I believe we should try to establish a truly comprehensive "Bill of Rights" for the mentally retarded, because even now the rights of the retarded are under attack all over the nation.

Year after year, a bill has been introduced into the Florida legislature that would permit doctors in state hospitals to allow mongoloids and severely retarded persons to die simply by withholding life-sustaining drugs. The author of the bill, who, incidentally, is a medical doctor, says that of the 1,500 retarded patients in Florida institutions, 90% should be permitted to die. "Why not let them die," says the doctor, "when the money for their care could be used for such good social purposes." "$5 billion could be saved over the next 50 years in Florida," he says, "if the mongoloids in our state institutions were permitted to succumb to pneumonia." The medical doctor who proposed this bill in Florida calls his bill "Death with Dignity," by which he means death with dignity for the *retarded*. I suggest that if such legislation were to be passed in Florida or any other state it would be death without dignity, according to the moral principles upon which this country was founded.

This is not, of course, a new idea. A number of years ago, a similar plan was put into effect. Doctors were told, and I quote: "Patients whose illness, according to the most critical application of

human judgment, is incurable, can be granted release by euthanasia." This was 1939, and it was signed by Adolph Hitler. Over 100,000 people died as a result of those simple instructions. The authority to kill was expanded to include millions of patients suffering from mental retardation, schizophrenia, epilepsy, encephalitis and a social disease the Nazis called Judaism.

Don't we know yet that this is legally unjustifiable and ethically unsound? Yet today, many Americans continue to judge people primarily on the basis of their intelligence and their economic value to society. A few years ago, Dr. Fletcher, a well-known Professor of Ethics at the University of Virginia, wrote an article on which he tried to define a human person. He listed a number of standards on the basis of which he defined who is human and who is not. His first point was that anyone with an I.Q. below 40 was not a human being and therefore did not deserve, let alone require, consideration as a human person. In his judgment, anyone with an I.Q. below 40 did not even deserve the right to life.

You may think his position is extreme. But I assure you it is not. So I say the time is ripe to propose a "Bill of Rights" (human and legal) for the retarded.

You will have your own ideas. Here are a few of mine.

First, there is the right to life. Any product of human conception that has the ability to live outside the womb, if given the necessary time to develop, should have the right to be born. The retarded person deserves the right to life, the right to be born, as much as any other human being. Obviously, this is

Eunice Kennedy Shriver is executive vice president of the Joseph P. Kennedy, Jr. Foundation.

not an absolute right. We all know that even the right to life can be limited. For example, we can act in defense of our home or our country, even if our action may bring death to another person. Yet the principle remains: the retarded should have rights to life equal to those accorded any other person.

Secondly, the retarded should have the right to an education in their own community. You are all aware of the class action suits in Pennsylvania, Alabama and Massachusetts, in which decisions were handed down demanding that the retarded — even the severely retarded — have a right to education and rehabilitation services.

Yet, it seems to me the retarded cannot wait for every state to bring such suits. Just as we have a Civil Rights Act to prevent discrimination according to color or sex, so we should have congress pass an Equal Opportunity Act to prevent discrimination based on intellect.

Third, the parent of the retarded child must have the right to a choice of care within the community. In most states, parents must choose a non-competitive state institution that is crowded, far away, old, expensive, lacking education, rehabilitative and spiritual opportunities and with little chance for a person to exit into a fruitful life in the community.

As you well know, the mildly retarded, especially the young, fare far better in the community. Commitment, voluntary or involuntary, of the mildly retarded is totally unjustified and leads to a serious loss of the common civil and human rights that can be fully appreciated by the mildly retarded. By such action, usually without due pro-

cess, the right to vote, to drive, to inherit and to make contract is lost. If the retarded inherits property, the institution even acquires that property to defray the costs of care. Even more frightening, the retarded has no appeal mechanism, and may be institutionalized *without review* for a *lifetime.*

Fourth, the retarded should have the right to work, mentally retarded persons can do many productive jobs even in our highly industrialized and technological society. The emphasis should be to fit the job to the person and not the person to the job.

Fifth, the retarded should have the right to a sexual and family life. Dr. George Tarjan, a foremost psychiatrist in the field of mental retardation, points out that the retarded are always the first people to be thought "surplus" by society, and the most available for "social action" and eugenic experiments. Indeed, surgical sterilization of the mentally retarded is permitted by statute in 26 states. In 23 of these states it can be performed without consent.

On the question of who shall and who shall not be allowed to have children, I am concerned with the logic that equates high I.Q. with desirable parental traits and low I.Q. with the opposite. Again Dr. Tarjan says: "We must remember that the tests of intelligence were originally constructed for predicting success or failure in school not in society . . . "Surely by now we should have learned not to confuse smartness with wisdom or humanity. Or have we?

We have learned that the age-old notions about sex and parenthood among the retarded must be re-examined. A recent study at a state institution, where the sexes were allowed to mix freely, states that the retarded are in general more responsible, more puritanical and more sensitive to rules of proper conduct in sex matters than normal individuals. "The extramarital conception rate of our women patients would have given pride to any college president or high school principal."

Sixth, the retarded must have equal protection of the laws. When the retarded are involved or suspected of involvement in crime, no statutes exist that deny them rights accorded to every citizen. Yet, in practical operation of the courts, the retarded offenders are frequently deprived of these rights. The facts are that the mentally retarded are three times as common in the population of Federal prisons than in the general population. Such data have sometimes been erroneously interpreted to mean that retardation is characterized by criminal tendencies.

In fact, however, these statistics show that the retarded individuals are less able than others to protect their legal rights. In a recent study it was shown that the mentally retarded, at the time of arrest, have far more frequently waived their constitutional rights against making self-incriminating statements. The retarded are easily cajoled into confession — 59% pleaded guilty compared to less than 10% in the non-retarded. They have waived right to counsel and to jury trial far more than criminals with average intelligence. Likewise, reduction of charge is far less frequent with the retarded. In 88% of the convictions, no appeal of judgment or sentence was made.

Competence to stand trial and to understand right and wrong are difficult determinations. It seems to me that the use of flexible criteria dependent upon the situation would seem desirable since each retarded individual and each situation varies enormously. Thus, the doctrine of "diminished responsibility" in the retarded would seem most appropriate. This doctrine states that the defendent is neither wholly responsible nor wholly irresponsible; it calls for recognition of an allowance for varying degrees of mental impairment.

Some of these rights that I have enumerated may seem extreme. But let me assure you the need for them is great.

Just ten years ago, the mentally retarded were automatically excluded from jobs in the Civil Service of our national government. That administrative rule was changed by President Kennedy, and today more than 12,000 mentally retarded persons are working throughout the government in hundreds of significant jobs. Last year alone more than 2,000 received promotions on merit. Several command salaries of over $8,000 a year. At least 300 were given awards for superior service. And one young man, a toolkeeper at New Mexico missile base, received an Army medal for courage beyong the call of duty in putting out a fire that threatened millions of dollars of damage to his base. Loyalty, love, dedication, and courage — these are values that the mentally retarded live by.

And so we are learning that, with the proper help and by any standards of worth, the mentally retarded have great value to our society. In their naive innocence, they believe us when we talk about love, trust and sharing. In their striving to be what they think we are, they are devoted, hard-working and trusting. In the courage with which they face their handicaps and disabilities, they inspire us all to a new standard of achievement.

Yet, we are far from being truly civilized in our response to those who deviate from our social and intellectual norms. We deal with these people as clients or cases, rather than as human beings. Somehow, even as we attempt to deal with their problems, a dehumanizing process takes place, reducing them from unique personhood to a collection of cold data in a case history. Then we lose the individual and deal only with the case history. If society cannot treat those who are different, does not society dehumanize itself?

Is it not the obligation of society, and that means all of us, to value and nurture, above all, the moral principles which teach us that all human beings are equal in the sight of God, that those who have the most gifts have the greatest responsibility, that, indeed, those with the least must be entitled to the most in a compassionate society, and that every human being must count as one whole person. Shouldn't we prize these moral values more than physical prowess or intellectual brilliance?

So let us reaffirm our dedication to the rights of the handicapped, the weak and the mentally retarded in our midst. Let us guard our society against those who would let the retarded die in the name of "mercy killing," or "death with dignity," or intelligence quotients, or economic efficiency. Let us preserve our philosophic heritage which stated that "all men are endowed by the creator" (not by the congress, the state legislature, or the supreme court) with certain inalienable rights." And let us be sure that for the retarded, as for all other Americans, these inalienable rights include the right to life, education, health and legal services, the right to love, the right to work, the right, in brief, to be fully human in a humane and compassionate society. ●

Personal Perspectives in Medical Ethics

RICHARD L. RASHKE

What do physicians and paramedical persons think the issues are in medical ethics? The NCW interviewed seven to find out — a neonatologist, a counselor, a neurologist, a geneticist, a cardiologist/researcher, a cancer patient social worker and a physician member of the National Commission for the Protection of Human Subjects of Biomedical and Behavioral Research.

We asked each interviewer four basic questions: What is the most significant ethical medical issue you face in your work? How do you make a typical medical/ethical decision? How do you resolve a conflict between your ethical values and those of your patient if there is a difference? What is the most significant ethical/medical issue in society today?

Other than a concern about the right of the patient to have a major role in his/her health care, the interviews — never intended as a survey — reflected different perspectives stemming from diverse disciplines, experiences and personalities. Here are some excerpts.

Editor

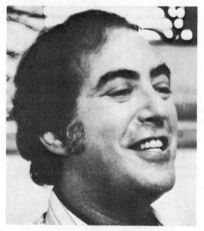

David Abramson, Neonatologist:
"Who has
the responsibility for what?"

Dr. David Abramson is a gentle man who often cries when a baby dies in his Georgetown University Hospital nursery, and who talks about living and dying more like a poet-philosopher than a physician.

As director of new born medicine, Abramson works with nine other neonatologists, thirteen fellows in medicine, thirty-seven resident doctors and Pam Bescher — a soft-spoken, empathetic counselor who helps parents feel comfortable with difficult decisions. On the average one baby a week dies in Abramson's nurseries.

Richard L. Rashke is Washington correspondent for the *National Catholic Reporter*, and a free-lance writer and photographer.

Abramson says the most important ethical medical issue he faces daily is: Who has the responsibility for what is patient care and the direction it takes? Abramson has worked out a formula with which he feels at ease. He reasons that two separate but interrelated decisions about critically ill babies have to be made. The physician decides what he thinks should be done based on available medical information and his own values. The staff reviews the decision critically. Then the physician tells the parents what he thinks is best and tries to get an informed consent. "That means you tell the parents completely what you think is wrong, what you think should be done, what the expected outcome is, what the common complications might be, what else might be done that you are not suggesting," Abramson says. "When you are convinced they understand that, then you're free to go ahead and get their consent."

Once the parents have made a decision, Abramson follows it unless he thinks it's unethical such as refusing permission for a blood transfusion. Then he goes to court. "I'll try to explain to the courts this baby needs the transfusion as a life saving measure," he said, "and that the parents are not behaving responsibly, and that the state should take away their prerogative to give informed consent and either appoint somebody else or take that responsibility on itself. The courts do not readily do this and that is good. The obligation of parenthood is very important and the court should take it away only with reluctance. I think the courts have behaved very responsibly in this area."

Abramson has found that getting an informed consent from parents — for example, to allow their baby to die —

is not difficult. "The problem is in medicine itself, especially with doctors who don't deal with critically ill patients every day," he said. "Death is seen as an enemy, as something to be fought, and not as part of life itself. The reality is that death is a natural part of life that needs medical management, and it is perfectly reasonable to want your patient to die. There's nothing wrong or bad about that. I think that's where the major problem lies. A lot of physicians feel that we should avoid death — that's the doctor's job. I don't view the doctor's job that way."

Abramson says a lot of factors go into making a medical life-death decision about a baby, but that what it really boils down to in the last analysis is — what is best for that child. "There's been a lot of attempts to pattern it, so that we can have some faith in the way physicians and society make this decision," Abramson explains. "I think each decision is individual. I don't think you can classify or group them. It depends mostly on your feelings that come from indefinable things. The way I handle it personally is, I do everything I can until I have enough evidence that, in terms of human outcome, I would be happier if I were unsuccessful and can say: I don't want this patient to live, I don't want him to get better, I want him to die, although I would never directly kill a baby . . .

"You have to consider what will happen if you are successful, providing you can prolong the baby's life. What will be the quality of that life? And that's a very personal question. I put it on a love basis. As long as the baby faces a life in which he can give and receive love, then it seems worthwhile. But you can't put that into a computer. Life is not a medical question. It's much broader, and it's appropriate for it to be nebulous."

Except in clear-cut cases, Abramson always feels torn when he has to make a medical decision on a baby's life. "One of the things I need before I make the decision is I have to feel good about it," he said. "So there is a built-in check that way. Another thing is basic unanimity among my staff. I use the staff as the final check that all the considerations that need to be made are made. There is no set list of considerations . . .

"In terms of playing God, I feel that in a very real way to take a sick and premature baby who obviously is going to die and to put him on respirators, intravenous support and computerized technology in order to have him survive is much more godlike behavior. It is really playing God to intervene when God obviously wants a patient to die. That's not playing God."

Abramson believes the most significant medical/ethical issue in society today lies in how the doctor and patient view their respective roles.

Ideally, Abramson argues, the physician's role is to help the patient do what he would normally do for himself if he had the skill. "If you get a little cold, you may take some medication, decide to go to bed and take care of yourself," he says. "But when it gets to the point when you don't know enough to take care of yourself, you go to the doctor. At that point, most people are still willing to abdicate their responsibility to take care of themselves and to say: 'Doctor, take care of me.' I think that's wrong . . .

"It has a lot to do with the fear of death. Rather than confront that fear and make responsible decisions, we are perfectly willing to have someone else say: this is what you have to do to get better, do it.

That's how the patient abdicates his role. Most physicians, until recently, shared this fear of death and they really needed the kind of love that comes back when you save somebody's life. That was a key part of the motivation in becoming a physician and the ongoing feed-in you need to keep up the crazy hours and concentration — the kind of dedication that it takes to be a responsible physician. One played into the other very well with such obvious bad results."

Abramson doesn't think educating medical students and physicians is the best way to clarify doctor-patient responsibility. "I think we might be better off in dealing with the people," he said. "Teach them what to demand from their physicians in terms of informed consent which is not only their legal right but their moral responsibility. They probably are less resistant to change than the physician group. If they come in and demand informed consent, the types of people going into medicine will change. The medical community has always been very responsive to what the people want. The major shaping force in American medicine is whatever the majority of the people want."✻

At thirty-three, Pam Bescher looks more like a college senior than the mother of a teenager. But when she talks about helping parents cope with sick and dying babies, she's more than her thirty-three years. Pam knows the games people play to protect them-

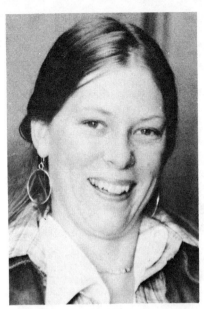

Pam Bescher, Counselor:
"Sometimes
I'll play devil's advocate."

have to go through, Pam continues — denial, sadness, guilt, anger — and it took several sessions before the father would talk about them. When it became clear to both staff and parents that the baby would never be normal enough to even feed herself, Pam began to probe how the parents would feel morally if the feeding were stopped and the baby allowed to die naturally. We talked quite a bit about their feelings. "Would they be able to live with their decision if they stopped caring?" Pam explained. "Often after parents have made the decision, we may wait hours or even another day until we are sure that's what they really want to do. If there are any questions, they would then have time to think about them. Often when they've made a decision and we feel pretty comfortable that's what they want, I'll play devil's advocate, just as the last check, because they're going to do that with themselves anyway. They're going to go home and ask: Gee, did I make the right decisions? I ask them: How do you think you'll feel next week, next month? And I let them know it's perfectly normal for parents, when they felt sure of their decision, to question it afterwards . . .

selves from their emotions. She and Abramson make a good team.

Take the parents of a child born with brain damage because of asphyxia (lack of oxygen), Pam begins. The baby's father is a white, Catholic blue collar worker who's embarrassed to talk about how it feels to have a baby daughter in intensive care. He sees himself as the strong husband protecting his wife from pain when he's really an insecure man threatened by his own emotions and hers. The mother is a nurse and more comfortable with hospitals, tubes and intense feelings.

There's a whole range of emotions parents of babies who aren't normal

"Very often we will encourage parents to come in and be with the baby if possible. Part of the process in counseling the parents is to keep the communication between them open . . . We encourage the parents to make a bond with their new born child. The grieving process cannot happen without the bond being made first. Parents will often go in and touch their babies and hold them or be there when the baby dies. If it's something like turning off the respirator, the baby will die very soon — within minutes. Then parents

9

are often present. That's a very individual thing."

It's not just the parents Pam worries about, it's how the life-death decisions affect the nursery staff as well. "We haven't really talked enough about how people on the staff feel when these kind of things happen in the hospital," she said, pointing out a weakness in the intensive care program. "We need some kind of network for people to help each other. These are very tough things to deal with. If everyone feels 'yes, it's time for this baby to be allowed to die,' maybe one nurse doesn't feel that way and doesn't say it. What does that do to her emotionally?" ✱

It's hard to even think of Dr. William Hawthorne as a cardiologist and physiologist. He loves to philosophize and only gets down to medicine itself when you press him for an "for instance."

Hawthorne, dean of Howard University's Graduate School, believes the laboratory is ten years ahead of doctors because the future of medicine is born there. As a research professor of physiology and biophysics, Dr. Hawthorne has spent many years in the lab. The absence of a consensus on ethical issues troubles him.

"While we spend a great deal of time in scientific approaches to problems of a biological nature, we have not spent an equivalent amount of time in the fields of ethics and philosophy," he said as he swiveled slightly in his executive chair. "So, we do not really have acceptable ways to decide what is moral and what isn't. Only recently have we begun to develop programs to get at this question. Until you decide that there even is a moral issue, you are left in that grey zone of what's right and what's wrong based on your own value judgments . . .

"We've improved our technology to the point of where it has forced this question on us. I think that is one of the

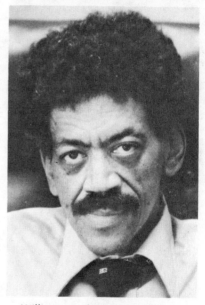

William Hawthorne, Cardiologist:
"Tampering with the evolution
of man's understanding"

great achievements of the technological developments. The advance itself forces you to consider issues which you would not consider. Without the ability to hook up patients to a number of machines, you never would have the question of who should pull the plug. That was forced on society well after the fact. The perplexing part of the problem is that if we now invoke rules and mores which do not allow us to get to the next set of technological advances – and therefore, the next set of moral questions – will we not be tampering with the evolution of man's understanding?"

When I asked Dr. Hawthorne what he thought was the most significant moral/ethical issue society will have to face in the next five to ten years, he said without a moment's hesitation: "Man-machine interface on health care delivery."

"As we look down the pike," he speculated, "more and more of the decision-making of therapy and health care will be part of computer systems and machines, pretty much like factories are today. The programming of these systems is going to require great care, and I don't really see that we have the tools to set up the human counterpart to that programming. In other words, technology may outstrip us so rapidly that it would be quite a problem to put back the professional input.

"More and more of the actual decisions are being made by the programmer, and more and more may be made by a programmer who does not have the professional skill of the physician, so that the quality control and the moral control of those decisions will have to be developed by the medical community in the process of trying to control their own machines."

For example, says Hawthorne, if you noticed an error in the payroll system of a university, how would you go about changing the program once it is set in cement? All you see are the checks, not the program, and that might not be enough to evaluate what is written. About all you can do is say there's something wrong with the program and it will take a long time before that filters down to some back room in the computer center. So the moral questions will be decided by a lesser trained member of society simply because of the technology of the system.

"It's a question of lack of control by default because the system is so vast," Hawthorne reasons. "Actually, the machine does not control man. What happens is that man programs a machine, but the man who programs the machine is frequently long gone and the machine, once programmed, is operating on another generation of individuals who have no impact on changing it."*

Dr. Robert E. Cooke is a member of the National Commission for the Protection of Human Subjects of Biomed-

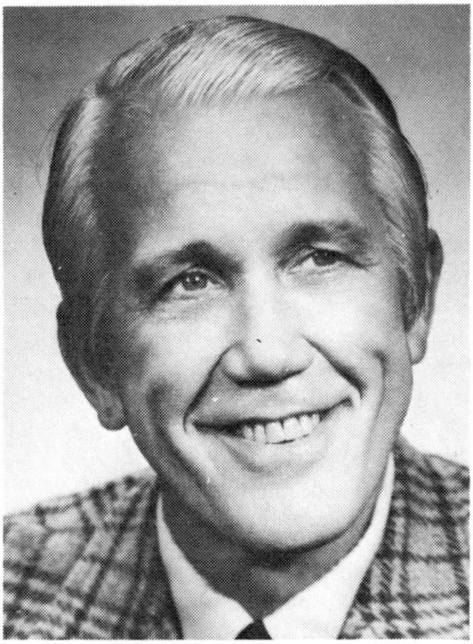

Robert Cooke, Researcher'
"The problem of free consent"

ical and Behavioral Research, and the Vice Chancellor for Health Sciences at the University of Wisconsin. For more than 20 years Dr. Cooke has conducted research on human subjects. I interviewed him by telephone.

The use of human subjects involves three basic ethical principles, says Dr. Cooke: do no harm, have the possibility of doing some good and be just in the selection of your subjects. "Justice is something that probably has been least considered in the conduct of research," he explained. "That means there should be no discrimination in the selection of subjects. For example, if I am studying a vaccine, then the subjects in the research should represent as much as possible those who will benefit from the vaccine. I would not find it appropriate to test the vaccine on children if it were meant for the general public, even though it might be administratively convenient to do so.

"It is true that the relative poor have been used in research, perhaps by default, because many of the people who attend large medical centers, which are located in the inner city, and who have participated in the experiments, are poor — not because there is willful discrimination against the poor, but because they were available. We need a greater sense of distributive justice. Prisoners, for example. I am reluctant to use prisoners as substitutes for the rest of the population unless we have clear evidence that the rest of the population will participate also."

Cooke believes there are several reasons for the great public interest in the use of human subjects today. The health care consumer has wised up, he says, and is beginning to demand accounta-bility from the professional. Then, there has been an enormous explosion in the research industry. Twenty years ago, the national research budget was in the millions; today it's in the billions. And finally, there have been a few really "monstrous misadventures" that have caught the public and political eye like the syphilis experiments on Tuskegee, Alabama, prisoners.

But Cooke denies that professionals are merely reacting to public pressures to regulate the research business. "There have been guidelines in Health, the Education and Welfare (HEW) research in particular," he pointed out. "They were quite thorough, detailed and comprehensive. But there were still some areas where all of us professionals had continuous concern. One such area was research on fetuses, children, the mentally retarded and the mentally ill. This is difficult since it involves proxy consent which is a complicated issue. The use of prisoners was another area, and some problems in behavioral and sociologic research had not been clarified. And then there's the concern about research not supported by HEW and not subject to its guidelines."

Another problem for Cooke is using human subjects without telling them they are participating in an experiment to insure the validity of the findings. For example, the researcher gives one group the drug to be tested and another a harmless placebo. "Many of us are concerned that so called deceptive research may not be justified," he said. "That does not wipe out the placebo. What it means is that participants should understand thoroughly that placebos might be used and they might get one. They would not know if they are on the drug in advance, but they would know that it is one of the possibilities. That's quite different from taking individuals and telling them they are receiving treatment, that it will help them, and then give them something that could not possibly help them."

Cooke said the most significant medical/ethical issue society faces today is the problem of free consent. First, he said, there is the non-consenting patient: the fetus, the child, the mentally retarded and the mentally ill. Even though these individuals as well as a future generation may benefit from the experiments, they pose a real dilemma for the researcher: Is the proxy ethical? But the root of the problem lies much deeper. "In general, I am pessimistic about what consent really means in the real world," Cooke reflected. "I have doubts whether it is possible to have truly informed and full consent. If I am told tomorrow I have incurable cancer, I am under great pressure, from within, to consent to damn near anything. So I am, in a sense, very vulnerable. Parents who have very defective children are very vulnerable. People in hospitals are very vulnerable. It is difficult to say when a person is making a fully free choice."*

Desmond O'Doherty is a conservative Catholic neurologist who speaks with a firm confident voice about the importance of the Hippocratic Oath. As chairman and professor of neurology at Georgetown University with 67 professional articles and books to his credit, he comes well credentialed.

O'Doherty sees Hippocrates' principle "do no harm" as the most significant ethical issue he and other physicians have to face day to day. "I have to make certain decisions about arriving at a diagnosis or giving a treatment," he says. "Some of the diagnostic procedures, done for the benefit of the patient, are a matter of judgment. And therefore, some tests have risks to them. I have to make a decision whether the risk is warranted in view of the purpose of the test. So that this idea about doing no harm becomes a very important one. In the case of a treatment, a similar situation arises."

On another level, O'Doherty sees abortion as the most critical medical/ethical issue society faces. "The whole deterioration of the medical profession is imminent if the medical profession, as a group, would succumb to the idea that abortion on demand was reasonable and had no ethical consequences," he says. "If we continue this way there will be no medical ethics left because if such a large thing in the Hippocratic

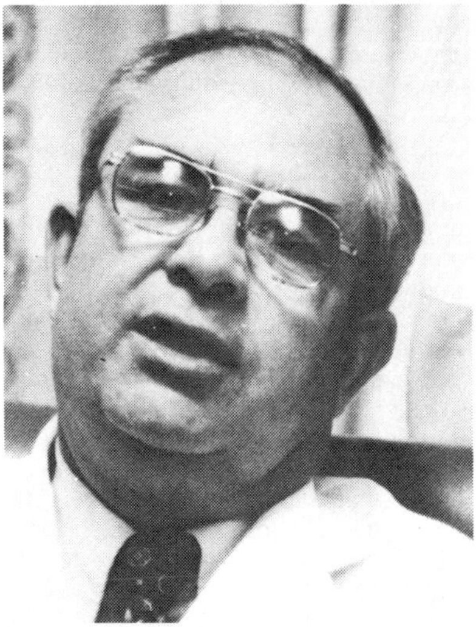

Desmond O'Doherty, Neurologist: "The courts have never been known for their wisdom."

Oath can be taken out, then the rest is is accidental, more or less."

What happens when O'Doherty comes into conflict with a patient over moral values? "I have a very easy recourse," he says. "I can withdraw. I can arrange for the patient to be covered by somebody else. All medical practice is a contractual relationship between a doctor and patient and either side can break the contract. If that were fully understood, we wouldn't have Quinlan cases and we wouldn't have other cases that go to the courts — a silly type of recourse . . . In the Quinlan case, for example, if the family felt the doctor was not sensitive enough to their particular problem, they should have discharged the doctor and allowed someone else to take over who might have been better disposed. I am a firm believer in the free practice of medicine — that patients have a choice of doctors and doctors have a free choice of patients. Where this doesn't work, then you have all kinds of abuse."

O'Doherty doesn't have much faith in the court as a mechanism to resolve doctor-patient differences on ethical matters. "The courts have never been known for wisdom," he argued. "Just look at society and you can see what havoc the courts can wreak on a civilization. I have no great feelings or expect any wisdom from the courts. They are only individuals giving judgments. To speak of the courts as if there is some great body of knowledge is ridiculous. It's one man giving a decision — that's what the courts boil down to. The second reason is a logical one. You have a man who is not trained in medicine or in moral theology, who is giving both a medical and a moral theological viewpoint in most instances."✳

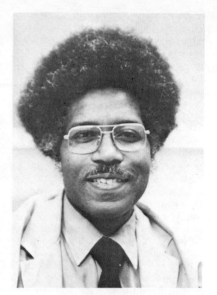

Robert Murray, Geneticist:
"A limit to our medical resources"

As a geneticist, Robert Fulton Murray studies and diagnoses inherited diseases. In the basement conference room of the Howard University Medical School where he teaches, Dr. Murray discussed some of the practical problems he and his genetic counseling staff face. Words flow easily for this articulate and sensitive researcher.

The thorniest, but not necessarily the most significant, ethical/medical problem Dr. Murray deals with stems from cases of suspected non-paternity. For example, in testing children for sickle cell anemia, Murray may find that a child has one sickle cell gene, making him only a disease carrier. Murray then tests the parents to make sure that both of them are not carriers because if they are, futue children may inherit the disease itself. In one out of 200 cases,

Murray says, neither parent is a carrier. Where did the child get the gene? There are two explanations: from another father or through a gene mutation, and there's only one in 100,000 chances of that. "Most often than not," Murray points out, "we have a situation where the biological father of the child is someone else. This happens often because so many woman are already pregnant when they are married, and they usually marry the man they love, the one they want most to be with and whose child they hope to be carrying.

"One has to deal with this without disrupting the family relationship and trying to be as honest as possible. On the one hand, if one is perfectly honest, one runs the risk of giving information — to the father in particular — that may end up in disrupting the family. On the other hand, one might be accused of being unethical or immoral by not telling the whole truth.

"We try to follow the principle of do no harm or of doing the least harm possible. We have come up with the formula of working most closely with the mother, discussing the situation with her to see if there was a possibility that this may have occurred. In some cases the mother may say: No, it is not possible; as far as I am concerned this is the baby's biological father and there is no way that anyone else could have been the father. Other times the mother will say there was a possibility but that she didn't think this other person could have been the baby's father. Then we work with her to decide how much to tell the father, particularly if there is some strain in the family already. Sometimes a child born with any disease, particularly an inherited disease, brings some stress to the family. The thing we want most to do is preserve the family

unit. So what we do is offer as much information as the father wants — that is to say, we offer the explanation of mutation as a possible cause (and it always is a possible cause), so we are not exactly lying. We stop there. Occasionally the father pursues it and says: Aren't there some other possibilities? Isn't there some other explanation? Then, if we have dealt with the mother and she feels it would be harmful for the family unit for the father to get the full story, we will generally try to stop there. We'll resist his effort at probing. But in the final analysis, he does have a right to the information. If he is insistent enough, as an occasional father is — most are not — then we will go with the further explanation or leave it to the wife to discuss with him because she is the one who may someday have to face whatever wrath he may have anyway. We make it very clear, if we do reveal what our suspicion is, that because we are suspicious and because non-paternity in our society is much more likely than mutation, it does not mean that it is not a mutation."

Only twice in Murrary's experience did families break up after the father found out he probably wasn't the father after all. In each case, the husband and wife were on the verge of breaking up anyway.

Another troublesome ethical issue Murrary has to deal with, but not too frequently, is related to abnormality in sex chromosomes. Hormones and/or an operation may be necessary to correct the problem.

"We had situations where a girl, who is a tomboy, feels more male than female as a result of her physical make-up." Murray explains. "She's kind of muscular and athletic. The child is thirteen or fourteen and her wish, as you detect it,

15

is to be a boy. The parents on the other hand, say: This is our little girl and if you are going to do anything, give her female hormones and do everything that's necessary to make her as much of a girl as possible. Whose wish-will should you follow? Some psychologists say you should do what the child wants; others say the child doesn't know what it wants — adolescents are so confused anyway."

How does Murray and his counseling staff of geneticists, family and social workers, psychologists, psychiatrists and endocrinologists handle such cases? "It's like a group decision where we try to take all the information available and put it together and come up with the best decision," Murray says. "But what we actually present to the parents are pluses and minuses. The story is never as clean-cut as we would like it to be. There might always be advantages in doing something in the other direction. So what we do is set up a plus-minus scale. Usually, we tend to favor the side where we have the most pluses. In some cases, the parents may want the other side. We leave it up to them unless it is obviously self-destructive."

And, as Murray points out, some decisions can be destructive. Take the male-like girl who was forced into becoming a female. When she saw her breasts developing, she had an emotional breakdown. Or the girl with testicles inside her body that have to be removed lest they become malignant. When she was told, against the advice of the geneticist, why she had the operation, it devasted her self-image. These cases are rare, Murray adds, but they do happen.

Murray sees the problem of resource allocation as the most critical medical/ethical issue society will have to face.

"In my own field of genetics," Murray says by way of example, "should we concentrate on finding ways to correct genetic defects, or try to find ways to prevent people who have genetic defects from being born or being conceived, or should we try to find ways of changing the genes of people who carry gene mutations? Or in the final analysis, if you are not going to do one or the other, how do you make a decision to apportion your money?

"Most people feel that if we just took more money from the defense budget or the Pentagon and put it into medicine, we could handle more of these problems. But it we took the whole GNP, we couldn't cope with all the possible medical problems. I don't know how you get people to face up to this." ✻

When Mila Tecala talks about cancer patients, words tumble out so fast that it's almost as if she's afraid she won't

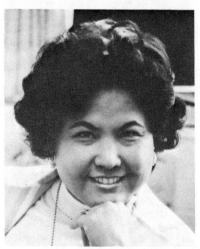

Mila Tecala, Social Worker:
"The patient is the primary focus."

be able to say all she wants in an hour.

For nine years Ms. Tecala, a Philippine social worker, has helped cancer patients and their families from diagnosis to chemotherapy to recovery or death. On the day I interviewed her in her tiny Georgetown University Hospital office, Mila had visited a 33 year old woman with a cancer that began in her breast, spread to her lung and spine, and finally ended up in her brain. "She was a stoic for a long time," Mila explained. "But then she called me on the verge of panic because suddenly her world fell apart. She is afraid she will lose control of everything, of her mind. Today, she was thinking she'd like to die and she asked for a living will.

"She sees herself as wasting away inch by inch. She was talking about getting off chemotherapy because she gets sick from it, vomits for three days. She gets so sick she can't even get up."

"Is it really worth that?" the woman asked Mila. "Can I enjoy a shorter life without having to go through that? Perhaps I will not live six months but then I will still be able to go to my garden."

The problem is the patient doesn't want to disappoint her doctor because she has a real fear of abandonment, or her family which clutches at chemotherapy as the symbol of hope. To complicate matters even more, her church is talking to her about a "healing."

"All of these are very confusing now that she's listening to her emotions," Mila said. "Somehow she can't put all of them together and somehow it all conflicts . . .

"It's not my position to tell her what to do. I always maintain neutral ground,

and in my work I make sure she knows what she is deciding on because it affects not only her own life but everyone's around her who must live with that decision — a decision she has every right to make. But before she makes it, she has the right to know all the facts . . . We talked about the advantages and disadvantages of chemotherapy, her hopes for the future. Tomorrow her husband and I and the doctor will talk to her about those things."

Mila believes the interference of the family in the patient's life poses an ethical problem. "Does the family have the right to hold that kind of bondage on the patient?" she asks. "That's where the patient is really having difficulty — putting together her family's wishes and hers. She is the type of person who would like to please everyone. And it gets very difficult because, at some point, she may have to disappoint her family since she can't continue to please them and continue suffering.

"I fully believe the patient is the primary focus of this whole battle with cancer. After all, she is the one to suffer. It is her life. On the other hand, the patient does not live in a vacuum. There are so many other things to deal with . . .

"There is always game playing going on in every family of cancer patients. One is always trying to protect the other. The problem with the game playing is that the patient is always the one who suffers. What I try to do is help them all understand that in some way they are not doing the patient any good by playing the game of either not telling the patient the diagnosis or by making decisions for the patient because they believe the patient doesn't really know what is going on. That assumption is very devastating for the patients. It is hard enough for them to deal with their condition; it's much worse when they are treated as if they can't make their own decisions. That just reinforces their fear of losing control. It makes the patient withdraw, give up and say: Well what's the use, I am no longer treated like a human being anymore, I am treated like a child.

"The family has to realize that, though sick, the patient can make rational decisions and that by taking the decision away from the patient, they are taking away an integral part of his life."

Mila believes the most significant medical/ethical issue society faces is "the decision to pull the plug."

"I think the medical profession is going to go through a great deal of rethinking in terms of what is death, how does one determine death or is it ever reasonable to decide on death," she said. "It's not just a medical question. Many other professions are coming into the discussion — philosophy, bioethics, even the clergy. I think that it is good that death is becoming an interdisciplinary decision. Hopefully, the patient will become part of that multidiscipline. After all it is his wife we are deciding on." ●

Moral Decisions in Medical Situations

LEONARD J. WEBER

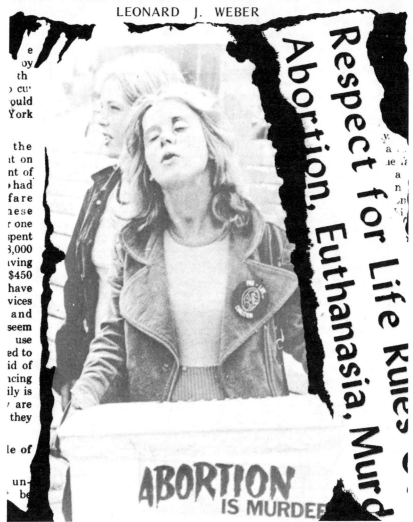

Respect for Life Rules

Abortion, Euthanasia, Murd

ABORTION IS MURDE

19

Some of the most agonizing moral decisions being made today in our society are decisions regarding what type of medical intervention is appropriate. As a society and as individuals, we wrestle with the question of the morality of abortion, we are unsure how much effort should be made to save the lives of severely handicapped infants, we are confused about what type of human experimentation is proper, and we are reluctant to decide what should be done for the dying. There is no way to produce unanimous agreement on these questions or even to guarantee that individuals will know their own stands clearly. The agonizing will and should continue; the questions are of such importance that they deserve nothing less.

Some efforts can, however, be made to clear the air. I would like here to focus on three dimensions of the problem of making moral decisions in regard to medical issues. The result will not be three easy rules for resolving these problems. The positions that need to be taken and the decisions that need to be made will probably be arrived at no more easily. Perhaps, though, these reflections will make us a little more aware of what is involved if sound moral thinking is to prevail in our decisions about medical care.

What would you do if you found yourself in a position similar to that of the parents of Karen Quinlan? What would you do if a member of your family was dying and there was no expectation of recovery? Would you request that no further efforts be made to prolong that life? Would you want to end

that life immediately if there seemed to be no other way to relieve the suffering? How would you make up your mind? For the sake of focusing this discussion, we will use this situation as our example.

When actually involved in a situation of this sort, some persons find it very difficult to make a decision at all. That is partly because of the tragic nature of the case. This may be the last chance to do the right thing for a loved one and we are not sure what is right!

Part of the difficulty, though, stems from the fact that we are not used to making decisions in medical situations. We are accustomed to letting the physician make the decision for us. Because modern medicine is so highly technical and specialized, we seldom have a basis on which to question a physician's diagnosis or prescription. We frequently let physicians determine our behavior; their recommendations are "orders" and provide an acceptable reason for not attending to our regular responsibilities (such as being absent from work). When it comes to medical care, there is no doubt that the physician is the one who makes most of the important decisions about what should be done.

There may be a tendency, then, to let the medical experts decide the question of whether to continue to try to prolong the life of a dying patient. That would probably be a mistake. Such a decision is primarily a moral decision, not a medical one. It is a decision that is based upon value considerations, whether the fight for life is worth it in terms of human dignity. Medical knowledge is necessary, of course. Those making the decision need to know what the chances are for recovery

Leonard J. Weber is professor of ethics at Mercy College of Detroit. Paulist Press has recently published his book *Who Shall Live?*

and only someone with medical expertise can supply that sort of information or evaluation. But the decision to continue or discontinue treatment is not based precisely on medical expertise, but on a judgment about the value of continued use of life-prolonging techniques.

Sometimes one hears a doctor say something like this: "As a physician, I would recommend an abortion if an unmarried teenager is pregnant." Such a statement is misleading. He or she is not making that statement "as a physician." Rather, such a recommendation is based on certain values that he or she holds, not on medical knowledge. A physician may be more familiar than many of us are with the nature and some of the consequences of teenage pregnancy and of abortion, but it is not medical knowledge that determines which actions and consequences are to be preferred.

Since the decision about whether to discontinue treatment is a moral one rather than a medical one, there is no reason why the physician should be the one who makes that decision. It is a decision that should be made by the patient himself, if he or she is capable of doing so. If the patient is not capable, the family should assume the responsibility. Ordinarily, they are the ones who can be counted on to know the patient's wishes and to be looking out for his or her best interests. A decision of this sort is best understood as the moral decision it really is if it is removed from the arena of professional medical competence and placed in the context of the family responsibility to care for one another.

The point is not that physicians have no role to play except to carry out the wishes of the patient and family, but rather that the proper nature of their role should be understood. Physicians sometimes make the decision to discontinue treatment in hopeless cases entirely on their own or with the presumed, though not explicit, consent of the family. This may be appropriate in cases where death is only hours away anyway, but in the more difficult cases, like that of Karen Quinlan, that would seem to be quite out of place. Physicians should not feel that they can never act without consulting the family, but their unilateral decisions should be the exception and not the rule. It is hard to see justification for a policy of letting someone else (whose values may not even be known) make a major moral decision regarding the life of a family member.

This, then, is the first point that needs to be remembered about making moral decisions in medical situations: such decisions are not to be left to the medical experts. We cannot expect to overcome some of the problems associated with medical-moral questions until we recognize clearly what is a moral decision and have the right persons assume the responsibility for making that decision.

There needs to be a close working relationship with the physician, of course. The first and most important dimension of the physician's role in this decision-making process is to provide all the necessary information about the patient's physical condition. He or she needs to explain, in a way that the family will understand, the nature of the condition, the type of treatment being provided, the consequences of continuing this treatment or any alternative treatment under consideration, and the consequences of discontinuing treatment. If the family is to make a wise decision, it is necessary that they have the proper information, which only the physician can provide.

The physician should probably also be asked to give his or her opinion on what should be done. That opinion should be listened to as the opinion of someone who, from experience, may have gained much wisdom regarding the best care for the dying. But it should also be seen for what it is — a moral opinion or moral advice and not in any way the authoritative word of an expert.

When the family has recognized its responsibility to make the decision and has the medical information it needs, it is only the beginning. Different people respond to the same information differently, depending upon the moral principles they have adopted and the way in which those principles are applied. As we continue to consider the question of the dying patient, we can become more aware of difficulties involved in moving from principles to a decision. We cannot here enter into the discussion of the proper principle on which to base decisions about human life. For purposes of our discussion, let us assume acceptance of the sanctity of life position and some of the immediate implications of that position as it has been applied to the dying patient situation.

Belief in the sanctity of life principle is a belief that human life is sacred and that its value does not depend upon a certain condition or perfection of that life. Since life is good regardless of the person's condition, there can be no justification for killing the patient directly (presuming that the patient is not committing unjust aggression against another). Euthanasia in the sense of directly terminating the patient's life is morally wrong, even when done out of compassion, because it is a direct and unnecessary destruction of a good life.

It has also long been held by defenders of the sanctity of life position that acceptance of death is not incompatible with respect for the goodness of life. We are not showing proper respect for the goodness of life if we neglect to provide ordinary care. But we do not always need to do everything possible to prolong life. Ordinary means of preserving life include all treatments that offer a reasonable hope of benefit to the patient and do not impose an excessive burden. Extraordinary means of preserving life are all treatments which do not offer reasonable hope of benefit or which do impose an excessive burden (such that other important responsibilities have to be ignored). We have a moral obligation to use ordinary means; we do not have a moral obligation to use extraordinary means.

These, I would argue (though there is no opportunity to do so here), are very sound moral principles on which to base decisions. But even with the acceptance of them in theory, we may be a long way from a good decision.

You may well have heard someone make a comment like this: "You can have all your moral principles and have your theoretical conclusions carefully worked out, but if it happens to you, you'll act differently." The suggestion is, of course, that in the heat of the situation principles will be ignored or that, when you are dealing with real persons, principles are too cold and unfeeling. And it may be true that the situation sometimes makes us aware of important dimensions of the question that we were unaware of earlier. But one must also guard against the danger of ignoring very important dimensions of the question precisely becasue we become overwhlemed by one particular facet of the situation. We may, for example, be so distressed by the almost constant suffering of a dying loved one that we become willing to do anything to put an end to that suffering, forgetting why we objected to mercy killing earlier. In an emotion-laden situation, we need to keep these moral principles in mind, not throw them aside. Becasue they have been developed with more than one situation in mind and because they have incorporated some of the wisdom of the ages, they provide the corrective lenses we need to keep us from viewing the scene out of focus. They provide the reasoned thought of many to balance against our own emotion. Emotion definitely has a place in morality, especially feelings of compassion and love, but it takes reasoned insight to understand the true meaning of compassion and love.

In many decision-making situations, there is a temptation to rewrite our moral principles on the spot because we feel more strongly about a particular point than we had earlier. We must be careful not to give in to such a temptation. There can be little hope for making sound moral decisions if we ignore guidelines as soon as we become personally involved. The danger of doing this may be especially great in medical situations because of the way that suffering affects us.

The second point to remember about making moral decisions in a medical situation is this: principles and guidelines are to be used, not ignored. We cannot let the pain of others and the feeling of compassion in ourselves lead us to ignore the moral teachings that we have accepted or ignore our own more calm reflections. Moral wisdom is not provided instantaneously in a situation.

We have outlined the guidelines for the care of the dying patient that we are using here and we have argued that these guidelines should in fact be put to use in specific situations. But the decision may not yet be made when we have gone that far. The application of moral guidelines is not always easy. Those who agree on a moral guideline do not always agree on its application.

According to the sanctity of life guidelines, it is wrong to directly kill a terminal patient. And probably all could agree that the administration of a lethal injection is directly killing. So the moral judgment in this case is not different from a logical conclusion: direct killing of patients is wrong; a fatal injection is direct killing; therefore, such an injection is wrong. But moral decisions cannot always be arrived at that easily. Those who agree that mercy killing is wrong many disagree on the question of whether turning off a respirator when a person cannot breathe without it is killing or not. The application of moral guidelines allows for much disagreement and, therefore, for much use of personal judgment.

This becomes especially evident when we consider the application of the guideline that extraordinary means may morally be withheld. What exactly is extraordinary treatment? The guideline helps a great deal, especially on the question of the hope of success. But what is "reasonable" hope? What seems to be a reasonable hope to me may not seem so reasonable to you. What about an excessive burden? It has long been argued by moralists that what is excessive for one person may not be excessive for another. It depends on how those involved are affected. The guidelines are very helpful, but they do not mean that there is no place for the prudent judgment of those involved. Such judgments are necessary if any decisions are to be made.

The ones responsible for making the decision (in our example, the family) should try to get what help they can so that their judgments are well made. As was indicated earlier, the physician is needed to supply the medical information. There may be others, too, to whom the family may want to turn. Some very good analyses of what constitutes killing and what constitutes extraordinary means have been done and, hopefully, a moral counselor familiar with these discussions will be available to the family in its time of need. But, many times, the decision will have to be made by the individuals involved; they will have to make the application to the specific situation through their own careful reasoning.

Thus the third point to be remembered when making moral decisions in medical situations: be prepared to make judgments and decisions on your own. It will not always be possible to find complete agreement even among those who accept the same moral principles. Moral guidelines are extremely important but they do not mean that there is no room left for the rational and moral judgment of individuals.

There are other points that could be raised about making moral decisions in medical situations. These seem particularly important and basic. As promised, these reflections do not make decision-making a whole lot easier. The agonizing will not be over. But if we keep some of these points in mind when we have to make the agonizing decisions, they will hopefully be decisions which reflect real moral sensitivity and insight.
●

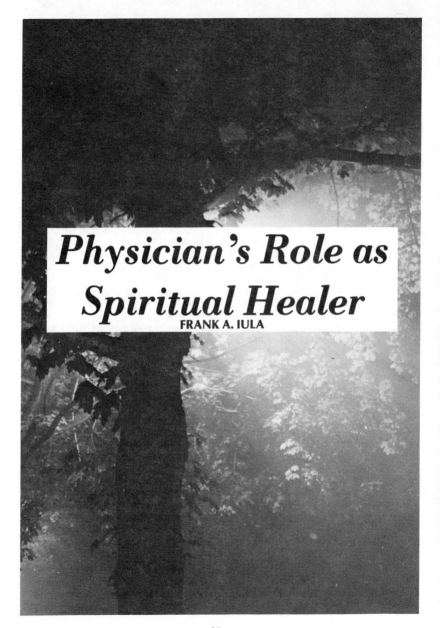

Physician's Role as Spiritual Healer

FRANK A. IULA

"If the Spirit of Him who raised Jesus from the dead dwells within you, then He who raised Christ from the dead will bring your mortal bodies to life also, through His Spirit dwelling in you" (Romans 8:11).

As a general practitioner for the past seventeen years, I have often been left with an attitude of futility and frustration concerning patients' needs. Many patients come to a doctor, desiring to be healed and cured of an illness which is almost impossible to diagnose, or is non-existing. Studies are diligently pursued and the final result is "everything is normal — all studies indicate there is no organic disease that can be medically proven." The response from the patient to this very authoritative and convincing statement is most likely to be: "But, doctor, I still feel ill. I can't sleep, I'm depressed, and I'm so tired I can't even do small household chores without feeling completely exhausted. My husband and children are disgusted with me. Doctor, please help me!"

This type of patient is a regular visitor in the offices of all practitioners throughout the world. What must our response, our approach be to those who beg and plead with us? Those who feel that the doctor is truly Christ, think that surely, somewhere in his "black bag" there must be a specific and special medication that will allow him to rise above the mire and live a life which is happy, joyful and peaceful.

Permit me to regress and flash back to 1970 . . .

Frank A. Iula, M.D., is a practicing physician who has become committed to the charismatic dimension of spiritual healing.

I have always been a church-going "Roman Catholic" who believed in God and sought a relationship with Him. I faithfully fulfilled my Sunday obligation, plus Holy Days of obligation, and placed my envelope in the collection basket each week. With all this, I felt there was an unfulfilled need in my life; a need not only for myself, but for others to whom I was endeavoring to administer in my medical practice. As a result of this felt need, I was led to a Charismatic Prayer Meeting and experienced, for the first time in my life that I could ever recall, the power of the Holy Spirit. I realized that Jesus Christ was alive and well, and wanted a meaningful relationship with me! I discovered, besides being Lord, He was also my brother. New vistas were opened up to me. I learned that the spiritual gifts talked about in I Corinthians 12 were truly given by Jesus, not only for the Apostolic Age, but for all succeeding ages. The Lord was giving me a new tool which to treat my patients in addition to the training I already had as a physician. I began to understand that I could be an instrument of His healing power. With this tool I could reach areas of my patients' lives that I did not have access to before.

Then, the truth struck me with a violent impact, the "voided" area which made me ineffective in administering to the needs of the "sick" — that is, those who were ill and had no organic disease; those who were sick and didn't respond to medications of any sort; this lacuna had to be filled, not by prescription but by a portion of God's healing love. These patients were crying out from the depths of their hearts because of emotional turbulence which had been revealed to us via modern psychiatry — psychology.

The feelings of just being "ill" didn't mean sickness — that is, sickness measurable in terms of organic diseases. We know that illness, due to emotional distress can surely cause organic diseases, such as ulcers, colitis, heart disease, etc. However, it could be independent of casual physical damage.

Professor Kelsey states: "As Jung stressed again and again, it was not he, as a psychiatrist, who achieved healing of a sick person. His task was, rather, to bring the individual to a source of healing found within the psyche, yet which seemed to come from outside of it, like a spring bubbling up into a little pond within the person."

I was totally convinced that the source of power of all healing was the Spirit of Jesus Christ, be it physical, spiritual or emotional.

If I could re-direct myself and bring into focus (in my own life) this Divine power by forming a personal relationship with my brother Jesus, I was convinced that I would begin to see God's power at work in my patients. I would be able to share His love and direct that love into the very hearts of my patients. The healings and changes of heart that were manifested as a result of this new, refreshing commitment, were healings that uprooted the cause of illness, brought them to a conscious realm and, once there, Jesus would heal each difficult area as it was revealed to the patient. I knew, too, that I must first use all the medical knowledge God had gifted me with to aid Him in our arrival at the truth. I was not to "sit back" and let Him do it all.

When a physician heals by means of drugs, therapy, etc., he is attempting to restore the patient to his original state of health. When Jesus heals, He does so in a deeper sense. The healing brought about by the Lord goes into the recesses of our subconscious mind, even as far back as our prenatal and neonatal areas which contain scarring within the person, resulting in not only a healing of the symptoms but of the total personality. Where, previously, a person may have been filled with bitterness, hate, egoism, jealousy, poor self-image, etc., these feelings were replaced with forgiveness, love and an improved self-image. There is a surge of well-being, ultimately turning us in a new direction. In short, there is an experience of "new life." There is a complete turn-about, revitalizing and bringing to life the Spirit within us that lay dormant. Difficult areas in our personal relationships are brought to light and healed through this new experience of the presence of the "Living God" within us. Man is reconciled not only to God but to man, to nature and to himself. The Old Covenant which was based on the observance of the Law is replaced by the New Covenant, epitomizing love above all else, a love that is divine in its source, and achieves fulfillment of the Law with a freedom never felt before. God allows us to rise above and go beyond the Law in our love for Him and our love for one another, giving us a deep sense of peace and joy that only He can give.

For the realization of a complete and total healing, we must bring ourselves into a genuine relationship with Jesus Christ. The only way we can do this is to present ourselves to Him as we really are. We must not appear before our Savior as a pretentious being, trying desperately to hide our true identity. We must not be afraid to come before Him "stripped" of the many masks we wear. If we are to be re-made in

Christ, we must be honest with ourselves and with our maker. This relationship can only develop when we call on the Spirit of Jesus to empower us with the trust that allows Him to cleanse and purify us. The Spirit-knit relationship that ensues makes the uniqueness of each person even more distinctive.

In seeking the aforementioned relationship, we are continually asking God to make us what we want to be or what makes us acceptable to our peers. Allowing Jesus to be Jesus is overwhelming proof that we want of Him what He wants of us. This is, therefore, the first and greatest giant step toward union with God.

The Spirit that gives us this union was not given to us "per se" to focus on itself but to direct us to another. That is, it shows us the way to Jesus and through Him to the Father. When Jesus speaks to us, enpowered by the Holy Spirit, power issues forth from Him and this power to heal is not aimed at our intellects, nor to change ideals. These "arrows of the Spirit" are aimed at the heart of the hearers and they are either accepted or rejected. At His touch, our whole being is asked to respond. The Spirit-borne words of Jesus always bring wholeness to all levels of incomplete existence (whether body or soul). Emphatically, Jesus heals the whole person. In Scripture, we read many accounts of Jesus healing the infirm. He never had to ask what kind of healing was desired, He simply gave what was needed . . . frequently to the astonishment of those who looked on.

In the Gospel of Luke (5:17-21) an account is given of a paralyzed man, presented to Jesus on a cot, for healing. Jesus, seeing the man's faith, said to him, "Your sins are forgiven you" . . . "I tell you, get up, pick up your bed and go home!" This is a prime example indicating to us that we are often "crippled" because of an emotional disturbance. This reaffirms that Jesus knows what we need even when we do not know ourselves. If we place ourselves trustingly into His hands He will reveal AND heal the areas in our life that are hurting us, according to His will — which is very often not our will.

A physician, using his God-endowed knowledge concerning the human system, is able to interfere beneficially with the ordinary course of a fatal disease. He does so by not violating laws of nature. Diseases which literally wiped out nations (diptheria, smallpox, yellow fever and typhoid) were eliminated by employing counteracting agents. Modern drugs, or so-called counter-acting agents, are found in our natural surroundings (penicillin — antiobiotics); rawolfia (for blood pressure); chemotherapeutic agents (for treatment and cure of malignancies); vitamins, etc. We can, therefore, state that modern-day treatment of diseases is extrapolated from nature and is considered to be God's way of aiding the physician to proclaim His glory. It is left to man's natural talents and intellect to probe and discover what God has placed before Him. The physician can be an instrument of God's grace.

Beyond the natural means of healing the sick (via counter-acting agents), there are modern-day healings that result through vigilant and concentrated prayer. These are known as divine or supernatural healings — the so-called miracle. No explanation, on a natural level, can be visualized or ascertained. Those who object to modern-day miracles say that they are impossible. Of course they are impossible to natural powers and that is what constitutes their significance. A miracle is evidence that a power above nature is at work. Whenever such a power is exercised it is evidence of supernatural approval.

Miracles which are stumbling blocks to some people are really stepping stones to divine faith and worship to others. Those who deny modern-day miracles and yet pray in private should give up the practice of the prayer of petition for this kind of prayer is appealing to a power above nature to aid one in some way outside the ordinary course of things. This is not said to discourage prayer but to show that those who believe in the Gospel miracles, but not in contemporary miracles, are inconsistent, unreasonable and illogical.

Admittedly, there are so-called "failures" in prayers for healings and a whole host of reasons can be set forth for this. It should be clearly stated and remembered that immortal life has never been promised with the healing of the mortal body. God never promised that we would not physically die. I do believe that many of us are actually offended and feel rejected because God did not listen or respond to our prayers in the manner expected by us. For example, when someone is seriously ill with a terminal disease and we prayed for a Divine healing and the person succumbs, we complain that God did not hear our prayers. True, He did not respond to our prayers in the manner we expected. God's promise to us was fullness of life and strength up to the measure of our natural life which does not end when we physically die but continues for all eternity with Him. Total and complete healing will be accomplished when we realize that this life is but a prelude to the eternal life promised by God.

Allow me to recount to you the medical history of a thirteen-year old, severely retarded male, a youngster named John, who is a gem to behold. He attends a special school and is able to walk and communicate with his family by gestures and facial expressions. He is somewhat toilet-trained and has a beautiful disposition and an excellent appetite.

In October of 1973, John had returned home from school when suddenly this happy, active child became very lethargic, subsequently began to vomit profusely and had fever and diarrhea. These episodes continued on a regular basis, once or twice weekly, each one leaving the child completely exhausted. The child's father, a physician, studied him very carefully; there seemed to be no answer to the problem. He was seen by a pediatrician, a pediatric gastro-enterologist, a neurologist and a hematologist. Many more studies were performed and all proved negative. The only possible answer given was that the boy's thermo-regulator system (an area in the brain that regulates body temperature) was "knocked out" by a possible viral infection. John's body temperature would soar to such heights that he would literally collapse from weakness; sporadic vomiting and diarrhea would then follow, sending him into a semi-conscious state. Still, there was no explanation. At one point, he was given four shots of antibiotics daily for ten days (for a possible salmonella infection, the existence of which was questionable). This effort was also futile. The youngster, who weighed only 40-42 pounds at his best, steadily lost weight and showed signs of dehydration and electrolytes imbalance. His parents, members of a Catholic Charismatic prayer community, never lost faith that God was in full control of the situation. The community prayed constantly for a healing and so did the parents. The Lord sustained both parents and youngster as these episodes continued for two years! Toward the end of the two-year period, John had a severe attack and was in a semi-comatose state at home. The father summoned the pastor of his parish, who is also auxiliary bishop of the diocese, and another priest-friend, for an anointing of the sick. Much to the parents' surprise, the bishop offered to confirm the child in the faith and did so. As the Sacraments of Confirmation and Anointing of the Sick were being administered, the mother and father of the child knelt, tearfully, at their child's side. Within them the prayer of relinquishment was taking place, and the father verbalized his prayer saying, "Lord, this beautiful child has been a gift from you to us. We relinquish him to You." At that very instant, the youngster, pale, limp and near death, jumped up from the couch, alert, smiling and happy. The bishop was astonished by what he had witnessed, and all those present thanked and praised God amidst tears and joy. The road back to a normal (for him), happy life, with few problems, was slow but steady.

Today, a little more than two years since the time of the first episode, Johnny is growing stronger, taller, and more alert than ever. He is one of the most joyful young boys in the school that he attends. Not much progress is expected in a child that is classified as severely and profoundly retarded. However, there are signs of progress in John's ability to communicate, feed himself, and recognize many of his needs. He is a perfect joy to behold —

I should know; this young, happy angel is my son! Yes — I believe in miracles!

The lesson here is that we must be completely broken before God can truly operate within us. We must be willing to "give up," surrender totally to what God knows is best for us. All of life is a gift from the Supreme Being, and at that point, when we can say, unequivocally, "I let go of all things," then God's total love and healing powers will be manifested in ways that are truly miraculous.

There are many illnesses which are beyond our scientific scope of understanding and we must ask God to intervene. Sometimes, the nature and source of disturbances that seem to be present in illness are beyond the limited confines of language. This is true because some of the factors involved arose during a period of individual development that occurred prior to language (e.g., infant, until time of speech, communication with the world is non-verbal; the infant is a passive receptor). Therefore, even well before speech develops in a child, the physical definitions of comfort, security, love, fear, etc., are laid down. Consequently, experiences in the infant stage (non-verbal) which may have been unpleasant, frightening, alarming have been suppressed and repressed, because of the inability to communicate these feelings. These experiences cause indelible scarring upon the individual and can remain throughout an entire lifetime, unless they are brought into the light to a conscious level and allowed to be healed by the Lord, usually through another person. This scarring manifests itself in a variety of symptoms (illnesses). The roots of these symptoms are buried deep within the development of the patient, inaccessible to his awareness, or the awareness of the physician.

Of course, we are also scarred in other areas of our lives, (infant, childhood, adolescent, adulthood) by impinging stimuli of rejection, lack of self-confidence, inability to cope with daily set-backs, frustrations and so forth.

We can conclude that a patient is a person with both illness and disease. The patient's response and improvement is related directly to the extent that both illness and disease are made better. Here we see the physician's role as not only a "curer" of disease, but also in his role as "healer" of the sick. The physician must at this point recognize his limitations. His armamentum of drugs can go so far in the restoration of a patient's health. When he arrives at an impasse — that is again, the organic nature of disease is healed but the patient still remains sick — he can call upon the greatest physician and healer to allow him to be graced with His divine gift of healing that He so graciously promised. Allowing this gift to flow through him the physician can administer to the patient (as an instrument of God's goodness and love) prayers for healing the whole person.

I have been blessed in that the Lord has used me as His tool in this area of joyful restoration of the sick to full health — mental, physical and spiritual. It is a delight, beyond comprehension, to see sadness give way to joy and weakness to strength.

God is a powerhouse of surprises. He never lets anyone down who believes in Him, always rescues us in the "nick of time." He snatches us from the throes of depression and sure death, to a plateau of heavenly delight — to enjoy a spiritual feast with Him, a feast like "no eye has ever seen" — savored with healthy portions of love — garnished with palatable heaps of joy and lavished with everlasting peace.

God is good — God did heal — God is healing and will continue to heal!
●

AN OVERVIEW OF MEDICAL ETHICS

CHARLES E. CURRAN

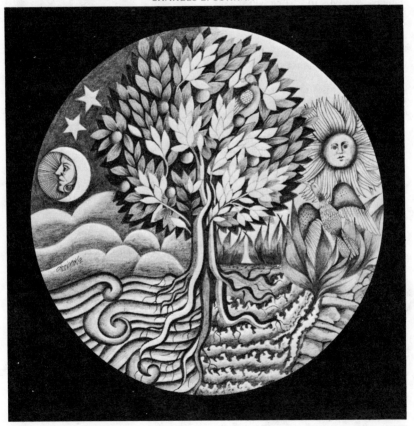

In the last few years no branch of ethics has grown more than biomedical ethics. An increasing number of institutes, publications and colloquia testify to its popularity. Questions of medical ethics are constantly raised in our newspapers.

I. HISTORICAL DEVELOPMENT

Such great interest in medical ethics is comparatively new. From the very beginning there have always been codes of ethics for medical practitioners, but

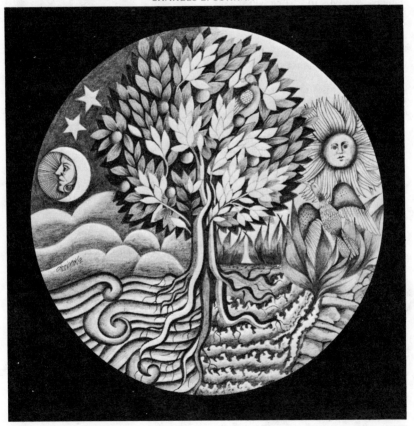

very often these were just repeated without any type of systematic elaboration and study. Until a decade or two ago medical ethics was primarily the preserve of Roman Catholic moral theology. Catholic moral theology's interest in the area is indicated in the number of books and articles that were published by Catholic theologians.

One must appreciate how recent are the developments that have led to the present state of modern medicine. Anaesthesia, for example, was first used successfully in Boston, Massachusetts, in 1846. Without anaesthesia most modern operations would be difficult if not impossible. In our lifetime there have been dramatic breakthroughs in our understanding of biology and genetics as well as in the development of medical technologies. In the area of human reproduction our knowledge until the seventeenth century was still based on thoughts existing before the time of Christ. Only little by little did science begin to understand the mystery of human reproduction, and it was only in the twentieth century that we came to know more exactly the process of conception and the time frame within which the male sperm is able to fecundate the female ovum.

Catholic authors even in the Middle Ages were interested in questions of biology and medicine. In the seventeenth and eighteenth centuries there were a few Catholic authors who wrote about modern developments in embryology and in human reproduction and about the obligations ·of physicians to their

Charles E. Curran, S.T.D., is professor of moral theology at Catholic University of America. He is author of *New Perspectives in Moral Theology* and other books and articles.

patients. In the nineteenth century there grew up a solid body of Catholic medical moral literature. Without exaggeration there are close to fifty volumes on various aspects of medical ethics produced in that century. Note such titles as *Moral Theology and the Medical Sciences, Pastoral Medicine, Physiological-Theological Questions, Morality and Its Relationship to Medicine and Hygiene.* This body of literature firmly established in Roman Catholic theology in the nineteenth century continued to flourish in the twentieth century as evidenced by the many volumes on medical ethics published by Roman Catholics in the United States right down to the early 1960's.

There is no corresponding body of medical moral literature among Protestant theologians nor even among secular moralists. The first significant work by an American Protestant was Joseph Fletcher's *Morals and Medicine*, first published in 1954. Meanwhile, the German Lutheran theologian Helmut Thielicke was also writing on questions of medical ethics. However, in the last decade there have been many books and articles by Protestant authors on questions of bioethics. In moral philosophy, ethicists especially in the United States showed little or no interest in specific questions in general let alone in medical moral questions until the last decade or so. Now institutes have sprung up throughout the country to study these questions; journals exist today which deal exclusively with medical ethics; an encyclopedia of bioethics is being prepared; medical schools which had been indifferent and ignored medical ethics now are incorporating such courses into their curricula.

What explains this historical development? Why were Catholc moral theologians practically the only ones interested in medical ethics for so long a time? Why has the interest burgeoned so much in the last few years?

Reasons for the interest of Roman Catholic theology. Obviously many factors explain the historical reality of Roman Catholic interest in medical ethics, but it is possible to point out some of these influences. First, in Roman Catholic thought at its best, reason was seen as a handmaid of faith and in no way opposed to it. The great medieval universities were sponsored by the Church which in theory boldly proclaimed that faith and reason can never contradict one another. (Unfortunately, at times in practice the Catholic Church lost its nerve and did not live up to this courageous assertion.) Many of the medieval theologians were also scientists as exemplified by Albert the Great, the teacher of Thomas Aquinas. Within the context of this ethos, Catholic theology was interested in biology and medicine and their relationship to theology and ethics.

Secondly, Catholic theology, unlike Protestant theology, stressed the importance and significance of works. Theologies which emphasized faith alone would not give as much importance to the morality of particular actions. Catholic moral theology, as contrasted with Protestant theological ethics, developed a comparatively exhaustive and minute consideration of human acts in its attempt to determine the morality of human acts. Such a generic interest in human acts and their morality indicates why Catholic moral theology would develop an interest in the morality of acts connected with medicine as well as other professions.

Thirdly, Roman Catholic moral theology from the late sixteenth century to the time of the Second Vatican Council was primarily in the service of the Sacrament of Penance training ministers and penitent alike how to know which acts were sinful and to distinguish among the various types of sin. Such a narrow perspective hindered the full development of moral theology both as a guide to Christian living and as a complete, scientific understanding of the moral life. This approach, nevertheless, gave great importance to individual acts and their morality and considered the problems that would arise for people in their various professions including medicine.

Fourthly, some of the early interests in medicine especially in the case of embryology came in the context of Catholic concern for the Sacrament of Baptism. Since baptism is necessary for salvation even of the child in the womb, the whole question of baptizing a child in the womb became a matter of both theoretical and practical importance.

Why were not others as interested? All these factors help to explain the interest of Roman Catholic moral theology in questions of medical ethics and why by the nineteenth century there was a unique body of medical moral literature in Roman Catholic thought. But why was there not interest by other Christian theologians, philosophers, and doctors themselves in medical ethics? In my judgment the answer is heavily dependent on the very nature of medicine itself. Until a comparatively few years ago the primary and only function of medicine was to help cure the individual patient. The increased knowledge and the capability of modern medicine have raised moral dilemmas and problems which did not exist in the past. Until well into the present century the primary purpose of medicine was to cure, restore to health, and care for those who were sick and dying. In this context the fundamental moral axiom was enunciated — no harm is to be done to the patient.

Ethical problems and dilemmas were comparatively few in the context of the older understanding and practice of medicine. Treatments, medicines and operations were medically justified in terms of the good of the individual patient. Conflicts between medicine and ethics rarely existed because the ultimate ethical norm was the same — a medical procedure of any type is justified if it is for the good of the individual. To justify most medical operations Roman Catholic moral theology employed the principle of totality according to which a part could be sacrificed for the good of the whole. Since the ultimate criterion of both good medicine and good ethics was the same, one could in a true sense accept the axiom that good medicine is good ethics. There was little or no room for conflict between medicine and ethics.

A study of the Catholic textbooks of medical ethics supports this analysis. Some significant questions such as consent, the obligation to tell the patient, and the use of ordinary and extraordinary means to preserve life were discussed; but the majority of the questions treated in Catholic medical ethics concerend questions of human reproduction. It was precisely in the area of these questions that Catholic teaching often ran into opposition from the thought of others.

The Catholic approach to human reproduction brought a tension into the question of medical ethics because according to this teaching the human sexual faculties exist not only for the good of the individual but also for the good of the species. If the sexual act, faculty and function (these were the terms of the Catholic analysis) exist only for the good of the individual, then there would be no real conflict. But the species aspect of the generative organs according to the Catholic teaching could not be sacrificed for the good of the individual. Thus contraception and direct sterilization were condemned. Today many Catholic theologians including myself deny such an older approach. A glance at the Catholic medical moral books indicates how much time and space were devoted to questions of reproduction.

In addition, problems also arose in the area of abortion. Here, too, the ultimate reason for the conflict was the fact that one is dealing not with merely one individual but with two. Consequently, moral dilemmas cannot be decided only in terms of the good of the mother. Obviously, these conflicts brought about by the question of abortion continue to exist today. It should be pointed out that until a few years ago Protestants and many other people in society along with Roman Catholics also generally rejected abortion so it was really not a burning issue.

The developing knowledge and technological capabilities of modern medical science have been the primary cause of raising many more ethical dilemmas than existed in the past. The ultimate reason for this stems from the fact that because of the possibilities of modern medicine our problems today no longer concern only alleviating pain and restoring health to the individual but there are many other considerations which also come into play. The remainder of this article will discuss the various questions being considered today and point out how they have often arisen becasue of developing medical and biological science and technology.

II. PROBLEM AREAS IN MEDICAL ETHICS

Death and life. Through modern technological developments medicine has at its disposal machines capable of resuscitation and of restoring circulation when breathing and the blood circulation have naturally ceased. The question therefore arises now which could not have existed previously: Should one pull the plug or refuse to use respirators in the first place even though they are readily available?

In responding to this particular question contemporary moralists have been able to learn from the Catholic theological tradition which acknowledged that one did not have to use extraordinary means to preserve human life. Extraordinary means were described as those means not commonly used in given circumstances or those means in common use which the particular individual in one's present physical, psychological or economic condition cannot reasonably employ, or if one does employ them they give no definite hope of proportionate benefit. The basic question always has existed, but the problem has become much more acute in the light of advancing medical technology. In the past people might have been faced with the question of whether or not to undergo a painful operation without anaesthesia. Today, however, most families sooner or later will confront the question about pulling the plug or never employing the respirator in the first place.

Catholic theology has traditionally condemned euthanasia because human beings do not have full dominion over their lives. God is the creator and giver of life, and we are stewards of the gift which we have been given. In the context of modern medical developments human beings exercise much more control and power over our lives and over our deaths than ever before. Also, one has to ask if there is always an absolute moral difference between acts of omission (failure to use extraordinary means) and acts of commission (positive interference to bring about death). These questions are now rightly being debated by theologians.

With the power of contemporary medical science to overcome disease and even improve the human condition, the question of the quality of human life has come to the fore. Through the alleviation of sickness, the overcoming of disease, and the prolongation of life, medicine has done much to improve the quality of human life. Through genetic engineering and manipulation even greater changes may take place in the future. Practical problems that did not exist in the recent past exist even now. Should surgery be performed on a baby to correct a grave malfunction if the child will be severely retarded or physically deformed even if the surgery is successful?

On a more theoretical level the quality of life raises serious questions. On the basis of the quality of life should the conclusion be drawn that some lives are more valuable than others? The basic Christian thrust admits the equal value of all, but the quality of life, if poorly employed, could be used to differentiate among various human lives. Christian and human ethics, in my judgment, under ordinary circumstances

36

(triage being an exception) shall uphold the basic quality of all human lives.

This raises the further question about the ultimate meaning and value of human life. Yes, medical science should try to overcome physical suffering, alleviate sickness and even contribute to the betterment of the individual and the race if possible, but the problem of suffering and evil must be faced on a deeper level. In speaking so much about the quality of human life, there is a great danger that our society will tend to forget about the weak, the handicapped, the aged and the poor. A very strong strand of the Christian Gospel testifies that these are the privileged persons in the kingdom of God. Ultimately in our technological and efficiency oriented society there is a danger of seeing the ultimate value of human life in terms of what one does, makes or accomplishes. A proper emphasis on improving the quality of human life and human existence must never lead to lessened respect for the handicapped, the retarded, the deformed, the aged, the institutionalized and all those others who are most in need of our compassion.

Intimately connected with the quality of human life is the problem of the proper meaning and description of the human. The problem arises in many areas today of understanding what precisely is the normatively human. Some are proposing quantitative criteria such as a certain level of I.Q., but in my judgment such an approach is difficult to reconcile with basic Christian understandings. In the light of newer medical technologies new tests for determining death are being proposed. The problem of the human is especially acute today in the whole discussion about abortion. In our

rightful quest of improving the quality of human existence, there is always the danger that we will write off as not human those whom we deem to be too much of a burden for themselves or who, perhaps more exactly, create too much of a burden for us.

The individual, society and others. Until a few years ago there were fewer problems in medical ethics because the primary focus of concern was the individual patient. Now things have changed. Transplants illustrate how one individual can be harmed or exposed to risks in order to help others. A paired organ is taken from one person and given to another in order that the second might live. Without modern medicine the person would have died. At first some Catholic theologians had difficulty justifying transplants because the only accepted justification of medical operations or mutilations (as they were called) was the good of the individual as incorporated in the principle of totality. But others, on the basis of charity or an expanded version of the principle of totality, were willing to justify transplants especially in the case of paired organs provided there was no disproportionate harm done to the donor. Now most theologians agree that there are limits to what one can do for another and great problems exist when the donor is a child who cannot freely and fully consent. Is the parent able to give consent for the child in such a case?

The almost miraculous progress of contemporary medicine would have been impossible without experimentation, but experimentation raises significant moral questions. The primary concern of the experimenter is not the good of the individual, but rather the individual is exposed to harm or risk for the good of others, or of society or of medical progress in general. At the very minimum, informed consent on the part of the subject is required for any experimentation to be justified. The person who volunteers for medical experimentation is more than an object, for the volunteer enters in a fully human way with the scientists in the quest for greater human knowledge resulting in good for others.

The current medical moral literature abounds in discussions about the nature of informed consent and the practical ways of safeguarding it in the context of modern medicine. Above all, special problems exist for those whose freedom is limited or even nonexistent — children, prisoners, institutionalized persons. These people often form the best control group from the viewpoint of scientific experimentation, but one must be very careful about abusing their freedom. Even though scientific progress might suffer there are times when a "no" must be said to scientific possibilities in the name of a Christian and truly human understanding of morality. Even for the average person a distinction should become more deeply ingrained in consciousness between the doctor-patient relationship which characterizes medical therapy and the researcher-subject relationship which characterizes experimentation. Not every "doctor in a white coat" is primarily interested in the good of the individual patient now being dealt with.

Somewhat the same tension exists in schemes for the betterment of the human race through genetic manipulation or genetic engineering as illustrated in the proposals of cloning which is accurately described as the xeroxing of human beings. But too often one forgets about those who might be sacrificed in the name of human progress. What about the mishaps and the mistakes? If one is trying to make a new type of chair, one can readily discard the errors; but what if you are dealing with human beings?

Another problem involving the individual and society concerns the use of societal or governmental persuasion or coercion or compulsion to force the individual to do what is thought to be for the common good. Nazi experiments on prisoners occasioned an awakened interest in medical ethics. The question often arises today in the context of population control. The freedom of individuals should be protected as far as possible, but freedom is not an absolute. In theory, compulsion and coercion cannot be totally excluded, but they should be used only as a very last resort. Especially in the problem of population control, there is a tendency to forget that the problem and its solution are ultimately multifaceted. There is a temptation of easily adopting simplistic approaches which see the solution only in terms of more and better contraception and/or sterilization and forget about the other needed remedies.

Priorities. A third area of medical ethical concerns which has come to the fore in the light of recent technological advances involves priorities. The question takes different forms. A few years ago a problem arose when there were not enough dialysis machines for all those suffering from kidney failure. Whoever was put on a machine would live; without the machine one would die rather soon. Who decided? On the basis of what criteria are people given the machines? One might think that the most reasonable way of distributing scarce medical resources would involve selecting people on the basis of rational criteria, but here one enters the tricky terrain of comparing one life with another. Ordinarily, the equality of human lives should be the primary consideration. In this light of insisting that all should be equal, the fairest criterion for decision making is based on random selection (chance) or merely on a "first come first served" basis after the medical judgment has been made.

There is a crucial problem of priorities within medicine itself, since there is only so much money, time and talent that can be invested. Sensational developments such as heart transplants attract great publicity, but should these be the number one priority of contemproary medicine? Human beings and not science should set the priorities. There is always the danger that the unusual, the esoteric and the adventurous will receive undue attention and funding. The Christian must always raise a voice in defense of the needs of the handicapped, the retarded, the institutionalized, and the well and frail aging.

Of special importance in the concern over priorities is the question about the proper distribution of health care in our society. From both the viewpoint of theory and of practice this has many significant aspects. It seems that there is a human right for every person in our society to have basic medical care. Justice in this case is based rather heavily on need and not on merit or the ability to pay for it. The basic minimal health care for all will naturally be different in different societies. Then there comes the very difficult problem of structuring the social system so that such fundamental health care is available for all people in our society. There are indications today that, whereas we have made gigantic strides in technology and medical advances, we have been fall-

ing behind in providing the basic medical care for our population. In addition, the astronomical cost of medical care has been a great burden on the poor and the middle class.

Human reproduction. Within Roman Catholicism there is still continued debate about the morality of contraception and sterilization. However, there also exist much broader questions that are discussed throughout the literature on the very meaning of human reproduction. Now there is much talk of test tube babies, artificial infecundation as well as artificial insemination, and cloning. Two extremes must be avoided. Catholic moral theology has rightly been accused, especially in medical ethics, of the danger of physicalism; that is, the tendency to identify the human moral act with the physical structure of the act. The moral and the physical aspects are not always the same. However, the physical remains a very important aspect of the human and cannot be neglected. The contemporary interest in ecology reminds us that the ambitions and pride of technological human beings have not always paid enough attention to the complicated ecological systems which exist in our physical world. In addition, the physical, as in the case of human reproduction, is also associated with many other important aspects and values such as the psychological. I will not absolutize the physical structure of human reproduction as something that is always and absolutely necessary, but I will not dismiss its significance as mere biologism. Moreover, in this whole area of artificial human reproduction there is the huge problem of the mishaps and mistakes which has already been mentioned.

Ethical questions of the profession. An area of continuing moral concern which is often neglected in contemporary writings might properly be called the ethics of the medical profession. What is the doctor's obligation to the patient? What is the difference between the doctor's relationship to the patient and the researcher's relationship to the subject? Problems of confidentiality and the keeping of secrets often arise. What about the obligation to inform the patient about the true nature of his illness? What about fee splitting and ghost surgery? Why is there a lack of doctors in our contemporary society? Has intense specialization really helped or hindered the general public? There seems to be a temptation not only for science itself to give undue importance to the esoteric and the unusual but also for philosophers and theologians to devote a greater amount of time to such questions. As a result, some of the ordinary questions faced by doctors in their everyday life are not discussed. One positive advantage of the traditional Catholic approach with its perspective of the confessional was to consider the problems faced in everyday life.

In conclusion, one cannot deny the importance of the questions being discussed in contemporary medical ethics. This article has pointed out some of the more significant problems we are facing. It is fitting and appropriate that so many people and institutions are now devoting their time, talent and treasure to such research. However one can never forget that there are also many other pressing ethical problems existing in our society.●

THE ETHICS OF

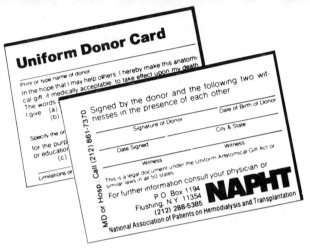

Uniform Donor Card

Print or type name of donor
In the hope that I may help others, I hereby make this anatomi-
cal gift, if medically acceptable, to take effect upon my death.
The words ___
I give   (a)
         (b)

Specify the or
for the purp
or education
         (c)

Limitations or

Signed by the donor and the following two wit-
nesses in the presence of each other

Signature of Donor   Date of Birth of Donor

Date Signed   City & State

Witness   Witness

This is a legal document under the Uniform Anatomical Gift Act or
similar laws in all 50 states.

For further information consult your physician or
                      P.O. Box 1194   **NAPHT**
                   Flushing, N.Y. 11354
                      (212) 288-5385
National Association of Patients on Hemodialysis and Transplantation

MD or Hosp. Call (212) 861-7370

As things get practical, ethics often get itchy. Some medical operations, procedures and techniques considered "impossible" only a few years ago are now quite possible and quite practical. Given the pragmatism so endemic to our American way of life and thought, some are likely to say: "If it can be done, it should be done."

The area of skilled surgical technique exerts a special fascination, if not awe, on the American mind. But this fixed

William B. Smith, S.T.D., is professor of moral theology at St. Joseph's Seminary.

concentration on continually improved means is not always accompanied by an equal consideration of carefully examined ends. Indeed, even to raise the question about ends and ethical means toward same involves the risk of being labeled an "opponent of progress." Yet it is often at this touchy crossroads that the ethical rub comes — here, one scratches the itch or scratches one's principles.

Some elements of the transplant question present few if any moral problems, but some other elements do. As more former "impossibles" become present "practicals," we would do well to heed

WILLIAM B. SMITH

TRANSPLANTS

the sound advice of Paul Ramsey that "the good things that men do can be made complete only by the things they refuse to do" (*Frabricated Man*, 1970), p. 123).

Along the same lines, the prescience of Pope Pius XII in medical-moral matters is again in the fore. The so-called "Harvard Criteria" for A Definition of Irreversible Coma refer to him (*JAMA* 205:88); all parties, oddly on all sides, in the tragic Quinlan case claim him; the author of a "save-or-let-die" ethic for grossly malformed newborns contends that his proposal is "implied" in the teaching of Pius XII (cf. *America* 131:8-9). My guess is that the teaching of Pope Pius is over-cited and under-studied because, in all the above instances, that Pope's discourses brought much needed nuance and many careful distinctions about means and ends which are too often overlooked by too many today.

In a discourse on "Tissue Transplantation" (May 14, 1956) the same pope urged an "intelligent reserve" which I think accords well with Ramsey's advice above, but is unfortunately absent from both unreserved endorsements and unreserved condemnations today.

Types of Transplants. Let us engage some of the aspects of the transplant question, beginning with the least problematic.

1. Authors refer to an "autograph" in which a part or tissue of the body is transplanted or resectioned to another place on the same body. Skin graphs in the presence of severe burns would be an example. This presents no moral problem apart from the question of risk involved. There is mention also of what some call a "heterograph," a trans-

plant between different species, e.g., from an animal to a human. Apart from transplants which might disturb physical and psychic integrity, e.g., animal sex glands to a human, there is no inherent moral problem here. Subhuman creation is ordered to man and the effort is geared to man's genuine advantage as man.

More usually, it is "homologous" transplants that are the center of discussion. Generally, these are of two kinds: static — from a cadaver to a living person; vital (*inter vivos*) — from a living donor to another living person.

2. The *static* transplant from the cadaver to the living person presents a few moral questions. This presumes, of course, that the deceased are treated with proper dignity, i.e., not treated as mere things, and that proper consent is obtained either before death or by legal custodian *post mortem.*

Perhaps the best known example is the cornea transplant. In this the eye is not transplanted but the clear, glass-like tissue which covers the eyeball is. The last few decades have witnessed great progress in this technique whereby the cornea can be removed and stored or preserved for some time in "eye banks."

Public awareness and public knowledge of cornea donation have increased through successful public education, much to the credit of several eye foundations throughout the country, the Uniform Donor's Card, and information issued by the National Kidney Foundation in New York City.

Similar to this would be the designated donation of singular vital organs *post mortem* (e.g., kidneys, heart). Clearly, vital organs necessary to sustain life, may not be removed until death has taken place (cf. *Ethical & Religious Directives for Catholic Health Facilities*, n. 31). About half the kidneys transplanted in the U.S. come from cadavers. A few years ago, such a transplant had to be done in less than two hours. Now, new technology has afforded a bit more time.

The facts and ethics of the above are generally free from controversy; however, the question about the definition of death and its statutory determination is not free from controversy. Some observers feel that elements in the transplant sector of the medical community seem interested in "advancing"the time of death to facilitate transplantations.

These questions should not be confused. The time of death and its clinical definition should rest on its own merits. One is either dead or one is not. One cannot be considered dead for special purposes (transplants) but presumably alive for other purposes (inheritance). It is important that the public understand this, for if the public should suspect otherwise the medical profession would suffer a great lack of trust. To this end, most transplant legislation together with our *Ethical & Religious Directives* (n. 31) state that in order to prevent any conflict of interest, the dying patient's doctor or doctors should ordinarily be distinct from the transplant team.

Another bit of the "intelligent reserve" of Pope Pius should be noted here — a caution against "utopian hopes." Perhaps, this is nowhere clearer than in the much publicized heart transplants. No one questions the technical expertise to accomplish this surgery; however,

the problem of immunological rejection still remains the big question.

Since Dr. Christian Barnard's first successful transplant on Dec. 3, 1967, we have all read about some of the more celebrated successes and even noted some anniversaries. Nonetheless, some seem inclined to read only the headlines while ignoring the obituaries. Long survival is the exception, not the rule; the average length of survival is less than two months. Much of the initial enthusiasm for this has tempered, again not because of uncertain surgical technique, but because the rejection problem remains. Kidney transplants are also not without problems; a successful "take" is about 50-50, with a 70% success rate among relatives, and the highest success rates by or between identical twins.

These cautions are not inserted to dampen enthusiasm or impede medical progress, but rather to temper the question with realism. Neither science nor morals nor patients are well served by unrealistic hopes or undeliverable promises.

3. The *vital* homologous transplant (*inter vivos*) presents us with the more complex moral questions, some of which have not yet been resolved to the satisfaction of all. While the basic outline is relatively settled, questions of detail and a consistent justification are incomplete. Here, again, a certain "intelligent reserve" is called for.

There is a history to the morality of transplants *inter vivos*. While some steps in that history are inconclusive, each step and each misstep is instructive. There is a subtle complexus of moral principles involved in the justification of *inter vivos* transplants, and that complexity should not be overlooked or ignored just to be "with it" or "against it."

First, we should recall, as Ramsey properly does, that this is the first time in the history of medicine that a procedure has been adopted and endorsed in which a perfectly healthy person is permanently injured in order to improve the well-being of another. (Our focus here is on genuine mutilations — the removal or excision of a non-replaceable part or organ. Here we are not concerned with blood transfusions and the like in which what is removed is almost immediately and naturally replaced. Our question is a positive excision which is not replaced.)

When such transplants became practical, theologians questioned how one could reconcile a directly intended mutilation of a perfectly healthy organ with the principle of totality. Concisely, the principle of totality is understood to mean that the parts of a physical entity, as parts, are ordered to the good of that whole physical entity. Thus, apart from the generative system, the intentional mutilation of a diseased organ or the repression of a function is justified when the good of the whole physical entity requires it — e.g., the common sense application of amputating a gangrenous limb because the health or life of that person strictly requires it. (If the same effect could be secured through less radical means, the less radical is, of course, to be done.)

In the transplant situation, the donor is presumably healthy. In those instances of double organs where the loss or excision of one is not a truly serious handicap, obviously it is not the integral good of the donor that requires and/or justified the mutilation; rather it is geared toward the well-being of the other, the recipient, who needs a healthy or properly functioning organ.

At first, some suggested that an "extension" of the principle of totality was required, basing this move on the moral unity of the human family. In this, human individuals are seen as parts of humanity, in the same way, or almost the same way, as individual organs are truly parts of one human individual. It was this line of reasoning, a revisionist understanding of totality, which was rejected by Pius XII. While noting that the purpose in this line of reasoning was to heal or at least to soothe the ailments of others, the purpose being both understandable and praiseworthy, the pope rejected as erroneous the method and argument on which it is based (above talk of 5/14/56).

This contribution of Pius XII is often misrepresented, especially by some who are anxious to dissent from *Humanae Vitae* by citing this as an example of papal backtracking. The pope did not condemn organ transplantation at all; rather, he properly pointed out that if organic transplantation were to be justified the principle of totality would not do the job.

At the time, competent moralists in the field did not misrepresent the papal clarification. The Jesuits Connery, Lynch and Kelly reasoned (c. 1956) that while the principle of totality could not justify organic transplantation, neither did it necessarily exclude it. They realized that some directly intended major mutilations for the benefit of another were based rather on the law of charity — e.g., the obligation of a mother to undergo Caesarean section for the benefit of her unborn child.

44

Thus, T.J. O'Donnell, S.J. correctly argues that while the principle of totality put some limitations on organic transplantation, the principle of fraternal charity to justify *inter vivos* transplants is not without its limitations also (cf. his *Medicine & Christian Morality*, 1976, 109-110). Therefore, apart from mutilations that would seriously and permanently restrict functional integrity, or risk loss of life, a sound and safe theological view is neatly summarized in our *Ethical & Religious Directives:* "The transplantation of organs from living donors is morally permissible when the anticipated benefit to the recipient is proportionate to the harm done to the donor, provided that the loss of such organ(s) does not deprive the donor of life itself nor of the functional integrity of his body" (n. 30).

The reader might wonder why this author has taken the long way around to get to the practical point of a viable justification for organic transplants. My purpose is simple, but not simply stated. Reserve in this area is not disapproval, but is, I think, required lest in the rush to be helpful we end up harming ourselves or others. Some of the mistatements of the middle 1950s are back in circulation again, notably under the title of the "expanded" principle of totality.

Again, with Ramsey, we should be careful about dismantling strictures against mutilation and self-mutilation. We should also be attentive to the moral reasoning presented for same, because it is now all too common to change names and words without corresponding changes in reality.

The so-called "expanded" notion of totality was first popularized by Bernard Haering and now seems to be supported by several authors: W. Reich, M. Nolan, C.E. Curran, and, apparently, R. McCormick (*Theological Studies* 36, 1975, 503-509). Quite often this "expansion" is shrouded in Haering's oft-cited "wholistic" view of man — apparently, a person's totality being his or her full dimensions and relations: economic, psychological, social, environment, emotional and physical. No doubt, an even fuller description of one's totality can be presented by any of the above authors. But, however "expanded," this is no mere change in words; it is a new and different understanding of the principle of totality.

Much of this is connected with the expectations of and subsequent dissents from the encyclical *Humanae Vitae.* With Haering's so-called "wholistic" view of man together with a revisionist version of totality, one gets a new and different form of moral reasoning — what Pope Paul VI described as "ensemble morality" (*H. V.*, nn. 3, 14). In this, individual actions — be it a contraceptive act or an act of mutilation — are said to find their moral specification not as individual acts but as parts of a bigger program, a wider ensemble of actions, the wholeness of a whole life project.

This, of course, is a novel way of saying that the end (whole life project; proportionate reason; neighbor's need for organ) justified the means (specific action in question). No one likes to put things crudely, and there are admittedly differences in approach, but most of these "expansions" of totality approach frankly, a rather get-the-big-picture view of morality with a broad-brush methodology in which the physical integrity of a human organism and its finality and function are reduced to mere adjunct status.

Totality renamed is not necessarily or at all totality redefined. Conventional Catholic morality argues that both the principle of totality and the principle of fraternal charity have acknowledged limitations. Pope Paul VI did not avoid this point but spoke directly to it "according to the correct understanding of the 'principle of totality' illustrated by our predecessor Pius XII" (*H.V.*, n. 17). The "correct" understanding is the one specifically cited in footnote 21 of that encyclical, which is the same exposition of Pius XII we have been following throughout this paper (5/14/56: *AAS* 48, 1956, 461-462; 45, 1953, 674-675). Several current justifications for the directly intended mutilation of a healthy organ — be it a so-called "wholistic" view of man, an allegedly "expanded" totality, or an ethic of proportionate reason for acting — are a bit facile when placed along side the "intelligent reserve" and needed nuance of authentic Catholic teaching.

Perhaps so much reserve is cautioned here that it might strike some readers as excessive and thus not intelligent. Let us focus some attention, then, on the particular area of kidney transplants. Some news-reporting registers a mild form of astonishment that there are not as many volunteers in this critical area as there are critical needs. Some writing is so couched as to make the reader feel a bit guilty for not having donated one of his or her healthy kidneys to someone in obvious and genuine need. The need is genuine, and the voluntary generosity of those donating is unquestioned. Fortunately, since July 1, 1973, the Social Security system now absorbs the lion's share of the costs in both transplant operations and dialysis maintenance. Still, the financial factor is not problem-free.

Although we don't like to admit it, the quality of medical care you get in this country depends very much on your ability to pay for it.

Nonetheless, nature, apparently, is superabundantly generous because two healthy kidneys have several times the capacity needed to maintain health. Even with that fact it remains inappropriate to speak of "spare parts." Public hesitation about donating a healthy kidney is not entirely misplaced.

First, we are talking here of a morally "extraordinary means," and no one is usually obliged to the morally extraordinary. One is free to do so, but not required to do so. Also, as regards the donor, he or she must be in good health, i.e., two healthy kidneys. The donation must be voluntary, i.e., truly free and informed consent. Being "informed" here certainly requires being appraised of the risks involved. Some risks are immediate — the operation itself is major surgery; some risks are remote — if the donor should develop kidney trouble in the future, he or she will have only one kidney with which to face that future problem. Finally, in a given instance,there may be reasons present for saying that a particular operation offers an unusually poor prognosis.

Thus, whatever the circumstances, and largely because of circumstances, I do not believe that anyone should be "hurried" or "pressured" or "emotionally manipulated" into a hasty or uninformed decision in this matter. Free and informed consent should be just that — free and informed! If there is public hesitation or uneasiness about being a donor, it seems to me that it is incumbent upon the medical community to clarify the realities and risks involved through sound public medical education. In my view, neither medicine nor morals is well served by anyone who oversimplifies what is really involved.

As surgical technique increases but living donors do not, more and more interest centers on cadaver transplants. As above, we presuppose treatment with dignity and required consent. When we speak of cadaver transplants we obviously mean *post mortem*. Generally, there is no problem here, but recent interest in the definition of death and a statutory determination of death have raised many questions.

Since some philosophy of life is embedded in every definition of death, it seems reasonable to maintain that a definition of death is basically, but not exclusively, medical, and a statutory determination is largely legal. Several states have already passed a new legal definition of death — I know of eight at this writing. Curiously, these new definitions do not all read the same way nor say the same thing. In itself this is something to ponder: if you are dead in California are you dead in Illinois? Some states have defeated similar legislation amid controversy — some of the objections being legal, some medical and some religious.

Even more curious here is that the widest spokesman group for doctors disagrees with the spokesman group for lawyers: the American Medical Association opposes what the American Bar Association proposes. While the American Bar favors a statutory definition of death, the A.M.A. meeting in December 1973 decided that such a definition is neither desirable nor necessary (*JAMA* 227:728).

More recently, the A.M.A. at its 124th annual meeting (Atlantic City, June 1975) and again at its last meeting (Dallas, June 1976) reiterated its opposition to a statutory definition of death despite considerable lobbying for it. At their 1975 meeting, the Tennessee delegation proposed that it was in the public. interest to cease artificial life supports in the case of so-called brain death, and, secondly, that it would facilitate the transplantation of organs in their best condition. The A.M.A. voted down this proposal.

It is important here not to confuse matters of fact with motives of faction. Death should and must be defined on its own merits, quite independent of the needs and wants of others, regardless of how noble or worthy those needs might be. A living human being turns into a corpse by and because of biological reasons only, and there seems to be something of an unholy hurry to rush that judgment, indeed to legislate as law what is not yet established as medical fact.

Much of the present controversy is presented in overly simple terms. It is said that the traditional determination of death — cessation of heartbeat and respiration — has been overtaken by new technology. Thus, we now need an updated determination, especially a consideration of so-called brain death. However many times the term "brain death" is repeated, it is not always accompanied with a timely explanation. "Brain death" as such is a generalization that very much needs specification; single aspects of this question require article-length explanation. However it is helpful to remember in this that the same A.M.A. House of Delegates rejected the proposition that "it is now currently medically established that irreversible cessation of total brain function is determinative of death" (June 1975). Thus, it is not now medically established that irreversible cessation of total brain function is determinative of death.

Morally, there is no religious axiom from which we can elicit a definition of clinical death. In fact, our *Ethical & Religious Directives* state: "The determination of the time of death must be made in accordance with responsible and commonly accepted scientific criteria" (n. 31). That statement is understood to rest on and incorporate the pertinent teaching of Pius XII (Allocution of Nov. 24, 1957; *AAS* 49, 1957, 1027-1033). Here again, the needed nuance of the full papal teaching should be noted: "In case of insoluble doubt, one can resort to presumptions of law and of fact. In general, it will be necessary to presume that life remains, because there is involved here a fundamental right received from the creator, and it is necessary to prove with certainty that it has been lost" (*AAS* 49:1031).

Thus, while there are ultimate questions resolvable only in philosophical terms, certain moral principles and presumptions do pertain here. The verification of the fact of clinical death depends largely upon the repsonsible and commonly accepted criteria of today. Therefore, when the commonly accepted scientific criteria are commonly accepted and endorsed by the *whole* medical profession — as distinct from interested *parts* of that profession — then would seem to be the time to consider legislation. To legislate as law what the A.M.A. will not endorse as medical fact seems to me quite premature and very unwise.

Other developments in this area also

cause some concern. As the differing states legislate different statutory determinations of death, what is being achieved is the direct opposite of what the A.B.A. set out to approve. The aim was to achieve legal clarification; the result is legal confusion.

Also some of the advocates of redefined death either choose very poor words to express themselves or they are working on a hidden agenda which they reveal only by mistake. A transplant specialist at London's Hammersmith Hospital is quoted as saying that the decision to switch off life-support systems for "brain dead" patients is made several times a day in British hospitals. "It is only when some poor fellow starts blinking his eyes as he is being prepared to have his organs removed that there is a fuss. With death redefined, there need be no fuss at all "(*Daily Express*, Sept. 23, 1975).

On February 25, 1976, Amitai Etzioni, director of Columbia University's Center for Policy Research, spoke to the American Association for the Advancement of Science about "cadaver farms." The "farms" would be equipped with machines that could keep human bodies artificially functioning as "sources" of such things as blood and vaccines. "The technical advantages would be enormous, but the moral questions are tremendous," he said. He noted that "farming the body" is possible through two developments: "a new definition of death," and "machines" that could keep the body running. As a gesture to social amenities he even thinks of a "ritual of parting similar to a funeral" to help the family along. Given what we now know are the realities of experimentation on aborted but living fetuses, these are not encouraging thoughts.

I do not raise these thoughts as absolutes but as questions, among others, which should be seriously studied and answered to the satisfaction of all before society rushes to judgment in this area. Willing one's corneas to an eye bank is fine. But let us be sure that intended donations *post mortem* really are *post mortem*. Making the back of your driver license an anatomical consent form may turn into something of a blank check. I submit that it is worth our time and study to discuss and review the presuppositions and presumptions of what is involved here — what is included and what is excluded. There are some rather aggressive interests in the transplant sector; the interest is welcome, the aggression is not.

"Harvesting organs" can sound rather agricultural and quite detached; however, with anything less than real certitude about real death, our legislatures could convert some of our fellow citizens into handy Army-Navy surplus stores just teeming with spare, but recyclable, parts. This is not likely to happen to a member of the Rockefeller family, nor to others if there is a lawyer or doctor in the family. But, having excepted that select group, there remains a very wide selection.

History does not suggest; rather history shouts and documents the fact that these kinds of hurried judgments always start small — such as with a small change in the law; or with a small slogan "they are dying anyhow"; or with a little loaded value judgment about a life or lives "devoid of value."

As we began, let me conclude with the view that "the good things men do can be made complete only by the things they refuse to do." It seems to me that it takes no small amount of "intelligent reserve" to see and to know the difference. ●

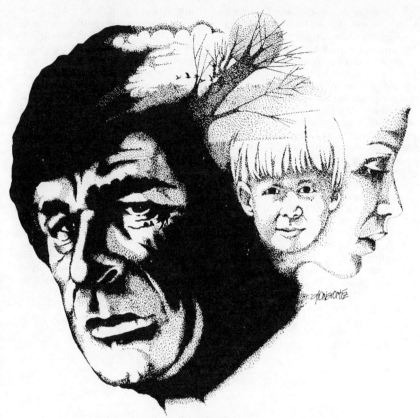

SAMUEL M. NATALE

THERAPIST'S VALUES
VERSUS CLIENT'S VALUES

It does make a difference whether the individual is considered as eager, curious, and trusting until specific experience in a given society and historical period lead him to be anxious, cautious and aggressive, or whether he is regarded as born with hostility, aggression, and fear which specific experiences may modify only to a limited degree in the direction of trust, sympathy, and interest.[1] Helen Merrell Lynd, *On Shame and the Search for Identity*

At a training meeting a few years ago, I found myself becoming increasingly uneasy for no apparent reason as students presented their diagnostic impressions and treatment plans. Progress reports followed during which cases were conceptualized with terms such as "Pathological Narcissism" and "regressive." Team discussions developed and aided in formulating a more effective treatment procedure. Each person contributed from his expertise and the outcome resembled a well orchestrated, multi-disciplined treatment plan that evidenced concern, care and a high level of training. A short time later on my way to the university, I heard a number of these same technical terms ("Pathological Narcissism" and "regressive") used again in informal discussion over coffee. This time, however, there was a notable difference — these same terms were now reflecting venomous disapproval. For example, "he's a real charcter disorder" or "she's always acting out." As I walked away, my former uneasiness focused and I began to understand why I was so uncomfortable during the earlier meeting. Although everyone was terribly interested in their clients, it was never clear what *function* the diagnostic descriptions served: were they *descriptive* or were they *evaluative?* Was a descriptive category cloaking a proscriptive notion?

This concern with linguistic precision is more than grammatical nicety. It is of the essence. Words used simply to describe a condition or a situation are necessary because they help the therapist and client to understand some of the elements/situations/reactions which they might expect regarding an emo-

tional illness (e.g., part of helping the chronic schizophrenic client is helping them to recognize the indicators that something is wrong again and to begin making contact with helping agencies, etc.). But labels that evaluate the person under the guise of description establish a pernicious goal which the client because of his docility/passivity may subscribe to (e.g., sexuality/bisexuality/ homosexuality). The therapeutic relationship deteriorates into a classroom exercise where the client is approved for "behaving" in the right manner or accepting a certain theoretical position about man (e.g., man is naturally aggressive) rather than another (e.g., man is naturally loving). Absent in this situation is any sense that the client is independent and has a right to explore, decide, etc. for himself in dialogue with the therapist.

Intervention and therapeutic technique are based on diagnosis and classification — at least they are supposed to be. In practice, however, the refinement and expansion of apparently reputable techniques of psychotherapy seems to have left untouched prior questions of considerable magnitude. If technique is based on diagnosis and diagnosis is being used evaluatively rather than descriptively, what are we about in our consulting rooms?

Any science collects, selects, and interprets data according to a more or less hierarchic structure. This is most appropriate in physical science, but when we are involved in a study that involves man without considering very specifically the issues and mysteries which surround him *qua* man, we have mindlessly transposed the technique of one discipline into another without considering the questions of values, appropriateness and reliability. We have degenerated from science to scientism.

Samuel M. Natale, S.J., D. Phil. (oxon.), psycho-therapist and university professor, is the author of *Empathy* and the forthcoming book from Paulist Press, *Pastoral Counseling.*

Science becomes scientism when methods successful in one area are transferred uncritically to another domain where its legitimacy is at best questionable. Psychology turned to established and more prestigious sciences to imitate them. But the established sciences were physics, chemistry, biology — each of which was developed within an implicit ontology suitable for nature but not for the human person. The natural sciences were never intended to study man as a person. One need not leave the realm of science to study man adequately. We need only to broaden science itself.[2]

In a flurry of activity we have generated models of man which are often in diametric opposition to one another. More alarming, however, is that the reliability and therapeutic *effectiveness* of the working model seems to be a function of the intensity with which the client and therapist subscribe to it. In short, if they *believe* in it.

The "belief" that has been so heartily and vehemently opposed when associated with religious affiliation now becomes the cornerstone of success for this new mode of treatment and "success" is often discussed in terms of the client's willingness to be "open" to the model imposed. The result is the frequently uncomfortable feeling that clients begin to respond to our expectations.

What precisely are we involved with here? Is the psychotherapeutic relationship an interpersonal event within which one is aided in exploring areas of concern, need and hope or is it, perhaps unqittingly, a classroom and testing ground for conformity to the values and ideas of a specific school of thought or therapist? It concerns me that so many clients are "classic ex-

amples" of Freudian, Transactional, etc., concepts. When this exactness pertains to the physical sciences, it is usually demonstrable and replicable, but when the same claims are made by a science of man and that science holds diametrically opposed models, something is wrong. Each system seems busily concerned with evolving techniques that will bring about the establishment of this "ideal" condition as defined by their theoretical stand. I don't find this particularly disquieting as long as the practitioners are aware that their model of man is tentative and that the "cure" frequently a function of prestige suggestion. (Prestige suggestion is the belief and subscription to the ideas and values of the healer and school of thought so that remission begins. The authority of the person "suggests" the cure and it happens.) Each school of thought is busy claiming "cures," but there seems to be a lack of concern for the establishment of our discrete observations into a holistic view of man. We seem to have forgotten that Freud, genius though he was, produced *one* model of man which was a distillation of 17th century mechanism, 18th century enlightenment, 19th century biology and a then growing notion of the unconscious. He has generated a model of man which has changed forever our understanding of motivation and consciousness — but it is *one* model. Each psychotherapeutic system claims its cures and remissions, rearranges values, emphasizes and ignores, selectively perceives, interprets and arranges. Each of these things is done within a prescribed context of beliefs about the nature of man as defined by the school of thought to which the therapist adheres. Bluntly, the therapist imposes his own values and selective interpretations on the client's world. It is difficult to find the observation and exploration characteristic of science in many therapeutic sessions. Often enough, the client is fitted into the theory. Theory is not expanded to accomodate the reality of the person. What we *believe* (as opposed to know) about the nature of man seems to provide the more usual framework for the explorations of our values and needs. Both therapist and client have values. In a healthy situation, it is the *interaction* and dialogue between these two persons and value systems that provides the vehicle for change. These value dialogues are essential because "it does make a difference" if we believe that people are naturally affectionate or that they are naturally aggressive. Belief effects choice, and we would intervene with our clients according to what we believe to be the direction of health. Nowhere is this more obvious than in the treatment of what is referred to as "sexual dysfunction." If we are going to ask our clients to trust us in a relationship where we hope to influence them consciously (and unconsciously) in the direction of growth and maturity, they have a *right* to know what we consider this direction to be. Even during treatment, a client's disagreement with our notion (and that is often what it is) is *not necessarily* "acting out" or "resistance" but may be the wisdom of his own accumulated experience. To expect the client to introject these values about the nature of man as the condition of improvement is an intolerable imposition. We may not honestly proclaim as concrete and certain that which is tentative and theoretical. Improvement should be a *description* of healthful changes that are agreed to by both therapist *and* client. Improvement is not mastery of behaviour approved by the therapist alone.

A review of the literature about patient improvement has been singularly disappointing and inconclusive. One conclusion is, however, clear: *improvement does not correlate* (correlation insignificant) *with the therapist's school of thought* (Humanistic, Freudian etc.).[3] Correlation is with the *personality attributes* of the therapist. In fact, improvement is a direct function of the personality interaction between client and psychotherapist, which provides preconditions for the exploration of the self. The values implied by any school of thought were useful only *after* the values of the patient, structured as he would choose to have them, were accommodated and accounted as primary. Sustained improvement was clearly a function of exploration of personal valuing systems and beliefs. Submission to any system was not the issue. Independence and the right to choose were.

If improvement (defined as increased personal freedom to choose) does not genuinely involve simple prestige suggestion or does not correlate with any school of thought or level of training, what, precisely, does it involve? As indicated earlier, counselling effectiveness has never been clearly established although improvement has been consistently associated with *certain counsellors*. These individuals performed consistently in a manner beneficial to the client. This consistency has been intriguing and has been the focus of considerable research.

When one looks to the characteristics of the psychotherapist, three qualities emerge. These were designated as "core conditions" and related to the theoretical formulations of Carl Rogers. They are described as empathy, genuineness, and non-possessive warmth respectively (Truax and Carkhuff, 1967; Truax and Mitchell, 1968).[4] *Empathy* was defined as the ability of the counsellor to grasp the meanings, needs and hierarchies of the client's world as if it were the client's own. *Genuineness* describes the ordinary meaning of the word implying honesty and openness (non-defensiveness). *Non-possessive warmth* was used to suggest a care for and valuing of the client and having as a goal the preservation of the client's dignity. A general summary of the research into these "core conditions" has been presented elsewhere (Natale, 1972)[5] and the problems of substantiating research into these variables has been voluminously attested (Truax and Carkhuff 1967; Goldstein, Heller and Sechrest, 1966)[6] Recent developments and emphasis on multivariate analysis have opened new possibilities and enabled us to isolate more or less accurately some personality variables. A study of film and tape recording of interviews has abled us to observe variances both *within* and *between* people. That is to say, although it becomes evident that certain consistent personality variables can be conceptually isolated for observation, it is also clear that different persons respond variously to different clients. We are faced with a Herculean task of trying to isolate variables concerned with client improvement for observation which can only be observed in process.

Valuable information has emerged. Therapists, rated high on empathy, genuineness and positive regard, displayed significantly different *use* of counselling technique prescribed by their school of thought. Therapists functioning at high levels of core conditions confronted their clients more often (Berenson, Mitchell and Laney, 1968)[7] Successful therapists were more likely to refer patient statements to their own lives, which adds to the sense of immediacy. A *human* relationship is clearly the vehicle of change. One final and urgent point: the research substan-

tiates that even with extensive training, therapists lacking the "core conditions" have little or no effect on their clients. In cases of severe deprivation of these conditions, client deterioration has been observed.

It seems then that we are once again squarely in the arena of the human experience: our models of man are significant and useful to the degree that we provide an emptying and clinical control of ourselves, which allows the client to emerge as the ultimately valued individual whose life and experience is unique and significant though inextricably involved with those around him. Our science gives way, not to mystery, but to respect, concern and a sense of our limitations.●

1.Helen Merrell Lynd, On Shame and the Search for Identity, New York: Harcourt Brace, Harbrace Books (paperback), 1969, p. 142.

2.Symposium on "Sciences and Scientism: The Human Sciences," Trinity College, May 15-16, 1970.

3.Frank, J.D., Persuasion and Healing, Baltimore, John Hopkins Press, 1961.

4.Truax, C.B., and Carkhuff, R.R., Toward Effective Counselling and Psychotherapy, Chicago: Aldine, 1967. and Truax, C.B. and Mitchell, K.M., "The Psychotherapeutic and Psychonoxious: Human Encounters That Change Behavior," In Feldman, M. (ed.) Studies in Psychotherapy and Behavior Change, Volume 1, New York: Wiley, 1968.

5.Natale, S., "Interpersonal Counsellor Qualities," British Journal of Guidance and Counselling.

6.Truax, C.B., and Carkhuff, R.R., Toward Effective Counselling and Psychotherapy, Chicago: Aldine, 1967. Goldstein, A.P., Heller, K., and Sechrest, L.B.: Psychotherapy and the Psychology of Behaviour Change, New York: Wiley, 1966.

7.Berenson, B.G., Mitchell, K.M., and Laney, R.: "Level of Therapist Functioning Types of Confrontation, and Type of Patient," Journal of Clinical Psychology, Volume 24, 1968, pp. 111-113.

MEDICAL NEMESIS
As Moral Education

EDMUND V. SULLIVAN

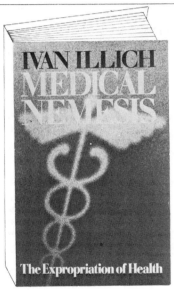

At a recent conference on moral and citizen education sponsored by one of the U.S. Government funding agencies, it was apparent that there is a growing interest in the whole populace on the topic of moral integrity. Participants at this conference discussed what implications this might have in the area of moral citizenship training. It was not apparent from the proceedings of this conference that there was anything fundamentally wrong with the American way of life or any of its sacred institutions. My own observation on this conference was that the *experts* in this area were sidestepping a deeper examination of the spirit of American life. It is very difficult for Americans to think or ponder that, in its affluence, North America has seemingly gained the whole world and in the process suffered the loss of its soul. Yet, in critical discussion of North American culture we find a growing suspicion toward large scale bureaucratic institutions and their inability to serve genuine human needs. Bureaucracies instead of building a human community tend to negate the personal, thus leaving the society in a soulless or personally alien state. There is an internal contradiction here, since the very presence of large scale institutions of a bureaucratic nature is justified by myth, advertising etc., on the basis of their positive contribution to the enhancement of the human community. The "medical bureaucracy" is a case in point since it justified itself historically as a healing profession, yet as we shall see from Illich's analysis, it tends to create the problems that it is seen to be solving. Our review of "Medical Nemesis" is within the context of moral education and this warrants some initial comments before discussion of the specifics of the book.

The title of the review is "Cultural Action and Problem Posing Education" and it is taken from the work of the South American educator, Paolo Friere. I will be advancing the notion that the "problem posing education" he outlines in his major works is in a true sense, radical moral education. More specifically, the notion of "cultural action for freedom" will be considered the *praxis* for moral education and one of the specifics of "cultural action" for a North American experience is a critique of medical professionalization.

(1) Friere's analysis of the South American experience is a creative attempt to establish a "pedagogy of the oppressed." The situation of this pedagogy is in transcending alienating social relationship which he describes as oppressor-oppressed relationships. *Cultural action* is a solidified action of people who are in an oppressed condition, attempting to liberate themselves from this condition by modifying their relationship with the world and with other persons. Cultural action is an action which links theory with practice (praxis) in a movement from a "naive awareness" of social action to a "critical awareness." *Naive awareness* does not deal with problems and gives too much value to the past and its inevitability while tending toward acceptance and mythical explanations. *Critical awareness* is a reflective cultural action (praxis) which poses problems about one's circumstances and is open to new ideas and new ways of looking at what was formerly considered an intractable state. Linguistically, education for a critical consciousness involves a *dialogue* with one's world and events, such that the person inolved in this dialogue is less prone to magical explanations for events in his world (i.e., mystification). This process Friere calls "conscientization" for which in North American

jargon the term "consciousness raising" suffices. *Conscientization* enables the oppressed person or group to reject the oppressive consciousness (naive awareness) which he is submerged in and to become aware of the nature of his situation in the "naming of his world." *Naming of the world* constitutes an act of critical judgment couched in a language familiar to the person coming to critical awareness. Critical awareness is a process (praxis) and not a final state representing a permanent effort for persons and groups to engender a program of awareness (i.e., education) which is situated in a history (bounded by time and space) seeking to achieve a creating potential in assuming *responsibility* for the state of one's world. It is in this context that I would label Friere's "problem posing education," moral education in its radical sense.

The "critical awareness" which Friere advocates is relative to each historical stage of a people and of mankind in general. Friere's own particular analysis has been in the context of the historical experiences of South America. Specifically, his problem posing education deals with a "conscientization" resulting from a literacy training program for Brazilian peasants. Content-wise he does not address the North American experience, except in a final section of his "Cultural Action for Freedom" (2), where he links the general structure of "problem posing education" to what he calls *Mass Society*. What then is "oppression" in a North American context? It is a condition of a "submerged awareness" (naive) produced by oppressive conditions inherent in the development of large scale bureaucracies in the North American experience. Submerged awareness is a *narcotic state* produced by large scale institutions in an industrial society. These institutions and their

Edmund V. Sullivan is joint professor of history, philosophy and applied psychology at the Ontario Institute for Studies in Education. One of his recent books is *Moral Learning*.

elite conception of what constitutes reality rob people of their ability to critically analyze their experiences of oppression. Professional advertising, medicine, law and schooling are just a few of these large scale bureaucratic enterprises. The development of "professionalization" produces an "elite" group (i.e., specialists or experts) who are seen as the superordinate definers of social reality in *Mass Culture.* A person in North American culture tends toward a state of *dependency* when he is confronted by the knowledge of the *"experts"* in the professions. Instead of "naming the world" (autonomy) there is a process of "having one's world named" (dependency) by depending almost totally on the judgment of experts. Therefore "school experts" define learning, doctors define sickness and health and lawyers define legality and custom. This whole process tends to rob individuals of their own critical abilities in defining their world and experience. In the context of North American experience, critique of the professions constitutes one aspect of a liberating praxis. It is in this light that I would label Illich's "Medical Nemesis" as a specific type of liberating praxis and therefore radical moral education.

To appreciate one component for a program in "Medical Nemesis" one has to realize that in the twentieth century, the medical profession has enjoyed the unparalleled adulation of the American public. Next to the U.S. Supreme Court Justice, the physician is ranked second in the public eye as a desirable occupation. It is one of many sacred cows that our culture dishes up to us in a porridge which discourages critical appraisal. Illich therefore plays the role of an "enfant terrible" when he brings a "problem posing" perspective to this sacrosanct enterprise. The problem is posed by the perspective which he brings to

bear on the possible ill effects of medical institutions. Consider the following startling statement: Unfortunately, the futility of medical care is the least of the torts a proliferating medical enterprise inflicts on society. The impact of medicine constitutes one of the most rapidly expanding epidemics of our time. The pain, dysfunction, disability and even anguish which result from technical medical intervention now rival the morbidity due to traffic, work and war-related activities. Only modern malnutrition is clearly ahead (pp. 21-22).

This statement is unnerving to say the least. Being a creature of modern culture I am initially disposed to view medicine uncritically. My initial personal reaction is to treat such an extreme view as the rantings of a crackpot or crank. When you read "Medical Nemesis" you may disagree with many things that the author says, decide that the author is a crank or a crackpot. To the contrary, you will be challenged on every page with evidence based on history and contemporary analysis for the thesis that Illich is advancing. Illich contends that his thesis is well documented and fairly obvious, but also well repressed. It is well repressed because we have internalized a cultural myth that the "Doctor Knows Best." The effect of our blind repression (i.e., submerged consciousness) of the technology of medicine results in *"nemesis."* "Medical Nemesis" is more than the sum of malpractice, negligence, professional callousness, political maldistribution, medically decreed disability and all the consequences of medical trial and error. Illich contends that it is the expropriation of man's coping ability by a maintenance service which keeps the user geared up at the service of the industrial system. In other words, the result of medicine is not more health but more medicine. This technology, as Illich defines it, is synonomous with the notion of *oppression* in the Friereian sense: This product is a package made up of chemicals, apparatus, buildings and specialists and delivered as medicine to the client. The purveyor rather than his clients or political boss defines the size of the package. The patient is reduced to an object being repaired; he is no longer a subject being helped to heal. If he is allowed to participate in the repair process, he acts as the last apprentice in a hierarchy of repairmen. Usually he is not even trusted to take a pill without getting a nurse. The medical profession has cornered the prerogative of administering most applications of modern science to health care. The argument that institutional health care (remedial or preventative) after a certain point ceases to correlate with any further "gains" in health can be misused for transforming clients hooked to doctors into clients of some other service hegemony (Medical Nemesis, p. 70). Illich's critical analysis is not centered on the physician per se, but rather, the whole interlocking network of medical professionals. He treats the development of this technology as a product of advanced industrial society. His critique of medicine is couched within a wider criticism of advanced industrial societies. Although there are many interesting side discussions on the nature of culture, the phenomena of death, etc., the main focus of the text is on three types of *latrogensis*. *latrogensis* is a technical term which simply means doctor-made disease: It is *clinical*, when pain, sickness, and death result from the provision of medical care; it is *social*, when health policies reinforce an industrial organization which generates *dependency* and ill health, and it is *structural*, when medically sponsored behavior and delus-

ions restrict the vital autonomy of people by undermining their competence in growing up, caring for each other and aging (Medical Nemesis, p. 165).

Although there are many aspects of Illich's analysis which are open to question and alternative interpretation, this work nevertheless provides a provocative analysis of an "elite profession" as perceived by most North Americans and is in the truest sense *"problem-posing"* in Friere's use of the term. It brings into question the *unquestioned legitimacy* given to modern medicine by simple fiat. When an institution like medicine lives off a fiat of this kind, the users of its wares may be considered in a state of "naive consciousness." I would contend that the reader of "Medical Nemesis," whether she/he agrees with him or not, is forced into a new level of consciousness (i.e., conscientization) concerning medical technology and its role in our lives. It simply forces one to face, at the very least, the possible oppressive side effects of one of the most sacred and mystifying institutions in modern consciousness. He raises within his analysis the question of medicine and its technology as a form of oppression and a denial of human freedom. This is a result of a process where: Each citizen tends to be placed into a patient relationship with each of several specialists. The number of patient relationships outgrows the number of people. As long as the public bows to the professional monopoly in assigning the sick role, it cannot control the multiplication of patients (Medical Nemesis, p. 77).

Now how can this analysis be construed as an experience of moral education? The position that I would like to see developed in circles where "moral education" is discussed is to see it as "cultural action for freedom." Cultural action is moral action when it is involved in the transformation of social structures which bind people to dependency relationships. Freedom is the activity and reflection (praxis) involved in liberation from oppressive structures, of which the medical profession from that perpsective of Illich is just one example. The focal point of a "moral education" relating to the medical nemesis could be in the careful and critical analysis (i.e., critical awareness as opposed to naive awareness) of the three forms of *iatrogensis:* the clinical, the social, and the structural.

Clinical iatrogensis is by far the most obvious and least disguised type of iatrogenesis. It is a damage closely related to physical symptoms and though difficult to detect, it is nevertheless the one most closely identified in suits of malpractice against the medical profession. It is more easily detected because you can receive the aid (for a fee) of another major bureaucratic profession (i.e., law) in your pursuit of this malpractice. Although I do not take this type of iatrogensis lightly, I would like to concentrate on the two other forms since they are more subtle and likely to be part of a submerged cultural consciousness (i.e., naive awareness).

Social iatrogensis is the addictive dependency of people on medical-care institutions. There are many points that Illich makes here worthy of consideration. Anyone who would attempt to reflect on this area in serious terms will realize the extreme dependency that he/she has on professional medical-care institutions. Reflection on and bringing to light this *dependency* would be part of a process of value training whereby an individual would be able to reflect on one of the major institutions in our culture which affects their lives. Illich's book is not for popular consumption because of his complex style of writing, but nevertheless it could be used by a teacher who is fostering a process of reflection on medical care. Moral reflection in the context of medical-care might likely take place in a health class. Illich's book could serve as one source of background and resource material for a *problem posing* education on dependency and medical-care.

Finally, *structual iatrogensis* is the loss of autonomy of the patient and the creation of a destructive dependency which takes away the meaning of significant events in one's life. Structural iatrogensis is assumed to be *intrinsic* in the values of the medical technocracy. It becomes a definer of the social reality (i.e., names the world à la Friere) which potentially robs individuals of the possibility of defining significant events in their own lives. *Structural iatrogensis* is indicative of a cultural malaise which sees the industry of medicine breaking with those social values and cultures, such as the acceptance of death, disease and pain, assumed to be in existence in the pre-industrial societies and which were capable of providing a meaningful system which did not make these events intrinsic to be technically removed. Illich's chapter on *death* traces the origins and history of the medicalization of *death*. Structural iatrogensis in the context of death is a process by which death is robbed of its profound interior meaning in the process of its being medicalized: The medicalization of society has brought the epoch of natural death to an end. Western man has lost the right to preside at his act of dying. Health, or the autonomous power to cope, has been expropriated down to the last breath. Technical death has won its victory over dying. Mechanical death has conquered and destroyed all other deaths (Medical Nemesis, pp. 149-150).

Illich trys to develop, under this heading, the thesis that a structural nemesis (negative consequence) is the increasingly man-made miseries which are by-products of enterprises (e.g., medical) that were supposed to protect man. The main source of pain, of disability and of death, "has become engineered, albeit non-intentional, harassment. Our helplessness and injustice are largely side-effects of the strategies for more and better education, housing, diet and health (Medical Nemesis, p. 155).

Illich's analysis of medicine under the rubric of these three forms of *iatrogensis* is provocative and *problem posing*. He comes to many conclusions with which I would be inclined to disagree, but I will not discuss these here because of the nature of this review. It strikes me that we in North America need more books of this kind which critically reflect on some of our sacred institutions. I wish the book was written in a literary style that would be acceptable to a larger public. Books of this kind are hard to come by because scholars who even talk about ordinary people end up by using a language that the mass public does not understand or appreciate. The potentiality for books of this genre for public service is obvious to my mind. They help the public to get a handle on a process of critical reflection of the institutions which profoundly affect their lives. I would put Nader's report on the auto industry, and Barnet and Muller's analysis of the multinationals in a similar category. I have tried to relate books of this kind to a form of radical moral education. In the context of cultural action for freedom they help to provide a reflective handle on some institutions which are profoundly affecting our values. It is in this wider sense that the subtitle reads "medical nemesis as moral education." ●

Friere, P. Pedagogy of the Oppressed. New York: Herder and Herder, 1972.

Friere, P. Cultural Action for Freedom. England: Penguin Books, 1974.

ADULT EDUCATION PROGRAM

BY SARA AND RICHARD REICHERT

GENERAL INTRODUCTION

The purpose of this educational supplement is to provide a practical plan for adult religious education. This plan will be based on selected articles from each issue of NEW CATHOLIC WORLD and will provide adult education programs for eight weeks.

Each session will be built upon key articles and will explode outward from these experiences, information, and group techniques.

1ST WEEK PROGRAM

A. INTRODUCTION

— AIM: To help participants clarify their own thinking regarding medical-ethical problems they are most likely to face in their own lives.

— Participants should have read — Curran's article.

— Materials: Copies of the article, blackboard or newsprint, writing paper, pencils.

B. EDUCATIONAL PLAN

1. (15 minutes) After providing copies of the article, leader asks participants to peruse it, looking specifically for all the kinds of medical-ethical problems the author identifies. As a participant finds one, he or she should mention it to the leader who writes it on the board or newsprint. Continue this until a complete list is developed.

2. (45 minutes) Form groups of six to eight each. Each group should appoint a secretary. Give the following instructions to the groups:

   a. Each person is to select from the list that problem he or she feels will be or has been encountered by him or her.

b. Participants then take turns explaining how they understand the issues involved in the problem selected and how they would or have resolved it in their own lives.

c. As each person finishes, the whole group attempts to identify the moral principles used in the decision.

d. The secretary records these.

e. When all have finished, entire group reviews the list of moral principles and prepares a report.

3. (30 minutes) Each group gives its report, identifying the problems most people feel they might encounter — or have encountered — and the moral principles used in resolving them. The leader may then wish to provide a brief summary.

2ND WEEK PROGRAM

A. INTRODUCTION

— AIM: To help participants evaluate the principles developed in this article by applying them to a specific problem.

— Participants should have read — Weber's article.

— Materials: Paper and pencils.

B. EDUCATIONAL PLAN

1. (5 minutes) The leader should briefly review the issues involved in the Karen Quinlan case. Participants can also be asked to expand on the leader's explanation.

2. (45 minutes) Ask all participants to place themselves in one of two groups: the group who are presently more inclined to think "pulling the plug" is rarely if ever permissible morally; or the group who are presently inclined to think "pulling the plug" is a morally acceptable solution in many hopelessly incurable cases. When the two groups are formed, give the following instructions:

   a. Each group should answer these four questions:

     i. What constitues death in your opinion?
     ii. What do you understand by the "sacredness of life"?

iii. Why aren't you "playing God" by your decision to "pull/not pull the plug?"
iv. Are you applying Weber's three principles?

b. Each group should prepare its report and select someone to present it.

Note: if the two groups are too large, smaller groups can be formed.

3. (40 minutes) Each group gives its report. The leader then facilitates discussion among all participants, allowing them to ask questions and challenge the conclusions of the respective reports.

End discussion by asking for a show of hands in response to the question: How many are now convinced "pulling the plug" is permissible? How many are convinced it is not permissible? How many remain uncertain?

Close with a few comments regarding the importance of Weber's third principle: BE PREPARED TO MAKE JUDGMENTS AND DECISIONS ON YOUR OWN.

3RD WEEK PROGRAM

A. INTRODUCTION

— AIM: To help participants clarify their thoughts on the question of the nature and possibility of miracles in our times.

— Participants should have read — Iula's article.

B. EDUCATIONAL PLAN

1. (First Alternative) Form a panel consisting of a representative of a local charismatic group, a medical doctor and a psychologist/counselor. The panel would present its views on the question of miracles. A general question/answer period follows.

2. (Second Alternative) Form a panel existing entirely of charismatics. Ask them to be prepared to give their views as well as any personal experiences they have had which might support their views. Follow with general discussion in small groups on the question: Do you think miracles can happen? Small groups then give their collective answer to total group.

3. (Third Alternative) Review the article briefly. Divide participants into small groups. Each group is to attempt to answer the questions:

a. How do you define miracle?

b. Given your definition, do they happen today?
c. If "yes" can you cite examples?
d. If "no" why are they impossible?

Groups regather to share results and discuss conclusions.

End with a prayerful reading of Mark 5:21-43.

4TH WEEK PROGRAM

A. INTRODUCTION

—AIM: To help participants attain a "critical awareness" of the role of the medical profession in their lives.

— Participants should have read — Sullivan's article.

— Materials: Poster board, felt pens or crayons.

B. EDUCATIONAL PLAN

1. (15 minutes) Leader and participants should review the main points of the article. Time should be spent especially on the key terms introduced like "naive consciousness or awareness" "critical awareness" and the like. Participants should be encouraged to give their immediate reactions to the article.

2. (45 minutes) Divide participants into groups of six to eight. Each group should be given a poster board with columns titled respectively "Oppressive Myths" and "Medical Service."

Through group discussion participants are to list under "myths" practices and attitudes which tend to keep us unduly dependent upon the medical profession or maintain in us a naive awareness. They might list such things as the saying, "The doctor knows best." In the other column they should list items which illustrate the authentic service the medical profession provides without making us dependent.

3. (30 minutes) Groups display and share their results. Leader facilitates discussion by asking for marked similarities or differences in the work of each group. Also ask participants to suggest ways in which the ordinary layperson can become less dependent upon the medical profession while developing a wholesome relationship with it.

Note: If a doctor or other representative of the medical profession is present, he or she should not participate but only observe. He or she will be given an opportunity to rebut the following week.

5TH WEEK PROGRAM

A. INTRODUCTION

— AIM: To continue the process of forming a "critical awareness" of our relationship to the medical profession.

— Participants should have read — Edmund Sullivan's article.

B. EDUCATIONAL PLAN

1. (First Alternative) Obtain one or more doctors to present a rebuttal to Sullivan's article and/or Illich's book. Show them the results of last week's session to help them prepare. Follow with a question and answer period.

2. (Second Alternative) If it is possible or inconvenient to obtain a speaker from among the medical profession, last week's exercise could be repeated. Simply replace medical profession with legal profession, education profession, banking profession or similar profession mentioned in Sullivan's article.

Allow members of the profession chosen to rebut if possible.

6TH WEEK PROGRAM

A. INTRODUCTION

— AIM: To help participants deepen their appreciation of the complexity of today's medical-moral issues.

— Participants should have read — Rashke's article.

— Materials: Paper and pencils, blackboard or newsprint.

B. EDUCATIONAL PLAN

1. (15 minutes) Review the article. Ask participants to identify the medical-moral issue each person interviewed stated as the most serious one facing society today. List these on the blackboard. Discuss each briefly to be sure the issue is understood.

2. Ask each person to select from the list the one issue he or she considers the most serious today. Groups are formed according to the issue chosen. For example, all those who choose abortion form one group. (45 minutes)

Each group then discusses and attempts to formulate a solution to the problem by way of a law they would introduce to Congress. If the problem does not lend itself to a law, they should attempt to apply a moral principle to be used when deciding the issue.

3. (30 minutes) Groups share results. Total group votes approval or non-approval of solutions offered to the problem.

Leader should conclude by reminding participants that some of these issues simply don't have clear solutions given our present development as a society. Or least they don't have easy or acceptable solutions.

7TH WEEK PROGRAM

A. INTRODUCTION

— AIM: To help participants clarify their understanding of the concept "informed consent."

— Participants should have read — Rashke's article.

— Materials: Paper and pencils.

B. EDUCATIONAL PLAN

1. (10 minutes) Leader should point out that several persons interviewed in the article observed the importance of "informed consent" in dealing with patients. Review the concept with participants.

2. (45 minutes) Divide participants into groups. Each person in each group is asked to recall an instance in his or her life where a doctor sought consent. Or they may prefer to describe the situation of a friend or relative. e.g., a woman with a history of problem pregnancy is advised that further pregnancy would be very dangerous. The doctor further advises tubal ligation as the safest process and seeks her consent. In the context of such a problem the group then discusses the resources other than the doctor to whom a patient may turn to develop an informed judgment of the situation and the medical course to pursue. Through these discussions a list of resources is drawn up by the group.

63

3. (30 minutes) Groups then share results of discussion. A complete list of resources is developed. Leader then re-raises for discussion the difficulty and the responsibility of both doctors and patients to arrive at informed consent.

8TH WEEK PROGRAM

A. INTRODUCTION

— AIM: To help participants clarify their responsibility and relationship to friends and relatives who are seriously or terminally ill.

— Participants should have read — Rashke's article.

— Materials: Paper and pencils, posterboard and felt pens.

B. EDUCATIONAL PLAN

1. (5 minutes) Leader should review key ideas in the interview of Mila Tacala.

2. (45 minutes) Form groups of six to eight. Instruct each group to discuss the problem of relating to seriously ill people. Ask them to share personal experiences. They may recall instances when they were patients or instances when they had to relate closely with the patient. From this discussion ask each group to develop a list of "10 Commandments" for relatives and friends of the seriously ill.

3. (30 minutes) Groups share results and attempt to develop one new set of commandments that integrates the various ideas listed.

4. (10 minutes) Seek several volunteers who would be willing to take this list and have it evaluated by medical and counseling personnel. When the list is finally edited make arrangements to have it published in the parish bulletin or similar communication media.